My Son Has Cancer

"A Mother's Courage to Hold God's Hand During the Storm"

Tawanda L. Davis-Hudson

Printed in the United States

My Son Has Cancer: A Mother's Courage to Hold God's Hand Through the Storm

COPYRIGHT

All rights reserved. Without limiting the rights under copyright reserved above. No part of this book may be reproduced, stored in or introduced into a retrieval system, or transmitted, in any form, or by any means (electronic, mechanical, photocopying, recording, or otherwise), without prior written consent from both the author, and publisher Tawanda L. Davis-Hudson, except brief quotes used in reviews. For information regarding special discounts or bulk purchases, please contact: Tawanda L. Davis-Hudson

PUBLISHER'S NOTE:

This book is a work of fiction. Names, Characters, places and incidents are products of the imagination. Or used fictitiously any resemblance to actual events or locals or persons living or dead, is entirely coincidental.

Copyright © 2018 Tawanda L. Davis-Hudson

All Rights Reserved, including the right of reproduction in whole or in part of any form.

ISBN- 978-0-692-13745-1

Library of Congress Catalog Card Number: In publication data.

My Son Has Cancer: A Mother's Courage to Hold God's Hand During the Storm

Written by: Tawanda L. Davis-Hudson

Edited by: Tradanius and Dr. Darlisha Beard

Cover Design and Layout: Dynasty's Cover Me

The devil rejoices when he thinks we are lost in despair. He laughs when we fall back into our wicked ways, but we put him to shame once we trust and hold God's hand with faith, courage, and hope. My story was written for those in a storm, coming out of a storm, or going in a storm. In other words, everyone need these reassuring words. Storms aren't designed to be easy, but they are well thought out and planned by God's perfect and divine will to make us stronger, and place us where He desires us to be. However, everyone that goes in a storm, won't come out to tell others about God's grace and compassion, but if your soul is aligned with His will, your Christlike qualities will display your faith, and others will see the God that existed in you. My son's journey will bless your heart.

In Loving Memory

Ja'Marcus Davon Davis, my dear son, I wrote this book in your honor based on your inspirational and faithful walk with Christ Jesus. Being merely 18 years of age, He blessed you to touch a countless number of hearts. My son, you will be loved forever!

A passionate dedication to my two baby boys, Baby Jay and Jorden. I only knew you in the womb, but you will always hold a special key in my heart. You boys are eternally mommy's little twinkling angels.

Big Mama and Aunt Shirley, I know you would be extremely proud of me. I am fortunate to have been nurtured by such amiable women. I'm thankful for each chastisement, for you ladies molded me to be a great woman.

THANK YOU

Acknowledgments

First and foremost, I thank God for putting my son and I in the storm. It was there, I learned to totally trust and depend on Him. Writing is one of my greatest passions, and I express great thanks to Him for my ability to write my first book. I thank you Lord for permitting me to give birth to a son that transformed my life forever. Ja'Marcus, I will never forget or stop loving you. You'll live in my heart infinitely. I am also grateful for my astounding husband. You encouraged and motivated me during my book writing process and I appreciate you. I owe a great debt of gratitude to my six children for keeping the noise level to a minimum, so momma could concentrate and write. I want to give a BIG SHOUTOUT to my eldest daughter Deshambra. Thank you so much for reading my book aloud from the beginning to the end...even though you wanted to be on social media. I LOVE YOU KIDDOS TO THE MOON AND BACK! I am greatly indebted to my baby brother, Tradanius and his wife Dr. Darlisha Beard. Thank you for proofreading my book. I owe you two BIG time.

I am appreciative for my Delmar Avenue Church of Christ family. You all were always there with kind words of encouragement. I extend a special thanks to the BEST minister in the MS Delta,

Dr. Billy Carl Moore. You equipped my son and I to fight this battle through the word of God long before the storm. I am thankful for you and your firm teaching. Sister Deborah Moore, words cannot meet the standards of appreciation that I have for you. The love you shown to us during the storm was awe-inspiring. You and Bro. Moore are the true definition of real Christians.

To my second church family, North West Church of Christ, I cannot thank you enough for your good deeds. West Oak Grove Church of Christ, I will forever be indebted to you and your splendid minister. Brother Matthew Myles, you were very instrumental to my son and me. Your phone calls and spiritual text messages helped me to get through those low-spirited days.

I want to extend a genuine and sincere appreciation to my Ruleville and Cleveland, MS supporters. You are simply the BEST! A heartfelt thank you to my Facebook friends near and afar. You all helped me to weather the storm, with your heart touching words of reassurance. Thank you for reaching out to my son and me. Your compassion will always be valued in my heart.

I could not leave out the world's GREATEST Make-A-Wish volunteer, Mrs. Bernice Wolfe. Mrs. Wolfe, you did her VERY BEST to ensure that Ja'Marcus' wishes came true. His Disney World trip was granted, but it wasn't possible, since he became suddenly ill. Mrs. Wolfe however, showered him with her presence and her earnest affection. I still have the personalized basketball themed blanket you gave him. You are outstanding!

I LOVE YOU ALL!

Introduction to the Storm

For a moment, imagine being told you have **cancer**. To walk in my shoes; through this dim storm, I need you to truly imagine looking at your doctor after you've been told "you have **cancer**."

How do you feel?

Weak? Nauseated? Stunned? Impassive? Flabbergasted?

These adjectives describe how I felt after being told my son had **cancer.**

Cancer is the most horrifying word in all languages. It is the most overwhelming word a person can digest. The word alone, hits you like a brick falling from the sky…one by one. Nothing to protect you. Identical to a deer on a lonely highway. **BOOM!** Just out of the blue, you never saw it coming. Now you're suddenly hit with a load of emotions. "Now what" is the question you ask yourself with great uncertainties. "Why me Lord" flows through your mind by the second, more times than you can tally. "Will I die" juggles through your mind, as anxiety fills your heart. All you have is faith.

The storm is in progress...

March 29, 2013, I walked into a bleak place in life. A place of worries, turmoil, rage and uncertainties. I dwelled in this gloomy place with an optimistic, but sorrowful spirit. I'd never been there before, and I have no desire to go there again, but for my child; I will.

"Your son has **cancer**" are the excruciating words the doctor pierced my heart with.

My mouth fell open in disbelief.

I pinched myself.

I knew this had to be a dream.

My brain gradually began to absorb the doctor's words.

"Your son has **cancer**."

This nightmare became my disturbing reality.

 My firstborn.

My pride.

My joy.

My heart.

MY SON HAS CANCER!

I was devastated, and nervousness defeated my body.

Within seconds a thousand pieces of my soul died.

My heart had been pierced like with a two-edged sword.

At that instant, I felt as if I carried the weights of every heartbroken mother on my shoulders.

This cannot be true!

What am I to do?

I am a mother.

I am Ja'Marcus' mother.

A mother's job is to help her child through adversities, big and small.

I was suddenly in a storm and I felt as if I had no direction.

How was I going to help my son during this intense moment in his life?

Was it even possible?

What would the outcome be?

I didn't know, but God did.

At the end of my son's 18-year journey on earth, I would sadly utter, "It's okay to leave me. I will miss you, but your momma will be okay." I would watch him take his last breath, just as I watched him take his first. As his mother, I will be there with him until the end, just as I promised.

Will I have the courage to hold God's hand during the storm?

Tawanda L. Davis-Hudson

Part I

In the Beginning

Chapter 1

In the beginning of May 1995, my life changed forever. I was unmarried, 18 years old and pregnant. Not only was I in the family way, but I was an embarrassed Christian. I had been baptized the previous year into the Lord's body, the Church of Christ. I knew what I had done was wrong, but I could not change it. My worst nightmare had come true. I was about to be a mother. I wasn't ready for this journey; therefore, I began asking myself questions that would affect my life. How was I going to walk into the Lord's house pregnant? What was I going to do with a child? I was a child myself. How was I going to tell my grandmother and aunts I was pregnant? I

knew they would be distraught for they had raised me better than my actions had shown. How would my baby's father react to the news "you are going to be a father, again?" Would he be prepared, enraged, or would he deny my child? Time would surely tell.

I was 3 months pregnant when I build up the courage to tell Big Mama I was expecting. Her reaction was not at all what I anticipated, for she peacefully said, "I already know." I was speechless. How did she know? My grandmother observed things closely. She used her "old school" wisdom to piece life together. Big Mama did not finish school, but she was smart. It was difficult trying to get anything over on her. She may not have said anything about a situation when it happened, but without a doubt she knew what was going on. She was an awesome woman, whom I admired wholeheartedly.

Big Mama is my grandmother, but, she is worthy to be called my mother. She loved and raised me as if I was her own. Everything a good mother does for her child, she did it for me. There was never a day I came home from school and didn't have a hot cooked meal. I did not wear fancy designer clothes, but she clothed me. She gave me everything I needed and some of what I wanted. She taught me what to expect about life. Big Mama was stern and she did not spare the rod. I now thank her for her firm discipline. She has gone to the moon and back for me on numerous occasions.

Big Mama's prayers along with the supplications from my aunts Shirley and Margaret, are the reason I am the woman I am today. I will endlessly love and cherish them. I am blessed to have been raised by such elegant women of God. They prayed me out of my mess in order that I could one day have a message. After a few weeks of acknowledging I was carrying her great-grandbaby, Big Mama began teaching me the do's and don'ts of motherhood. She prepared me to be a good mother to my child while he was yet in the womb. Being a pregnant child was not easy.

Every day was a struggle. I had to quickly mature for time was not waiting on me. I would no longer be "a little girl playing with a baby doll." Those were the words from my big brother Bruce, and he was right. I would soon be a mother with a real baby. Only the Lord knew how much teaching I needed on caring for a child. I had absolutely no knowledge of babies. I'd never babysat an infant before, and simply thinking about having the baby frighten me even more. "What had I gotten myself into?" were my daily thoughts. Everything was about to change and shortly a little one will be calling me "momma."

February 2, is the day my mother, Anna gave birth to my baby brother Tradanius, and my cousin Debra birthed her first child, Willie. Groundhog's Day must be a spectacular day of magic, for on February 2, 1996, I too was blessed with an extraordinary baby boy. Ja'Marcus Davon Davis was the name I'd chosen for my 5 pounds 15-ounces bundle of delight. He was a sweet and adorable baby. He didn't realize how much he'd touched my heart with a lifetime of love with just one glimpse. I refused to fail him as his mother. I promised him I would be by his side always. My grandmother and aunts were not happy about me having a child at a young age, but they were more than supportive. They loved Ja'Marcus as if he was their own. They were my main support system. His father of course, was lost in a state of "I am not the father since he does not have green eyes" syndrome. At 18 years old, I thought I'd be mad with him for his immature statement, but I was content with his thoughts of not being my son's father. I refused to let his immatureness affect my motherly duties to my newborn son. Ja'Marcus Davon Davis was going to be taken care of with him without him. My son was indeed in good hands; God and mommies' hands.

"Children are a gift from God"
Psalm 127:3

Embracing Motherhood
Chapter 2

The first years of parenthood were the toughest. After many mishaps, I swiftly learned babies were not born with guidelines. Being Ja'Marcus' mother was an unimaginable blessing. A blessing like no other, for he was the greatest gift I had received, besides accepting Christ as my Lord and Savior. The bond I had with him was insurmountable and unmatched. I wanted to be a good mother to my son. Being a mother of morals and virtue were not a factor, because with Big Mama and my aunt's help, I was **embracing motherhood**.

Taking care of an infant was hard work. I had to sleep when the baby slept and eat when he ate. I scheduled my days, so I would stay of sound mind. I would wake up at 6'oclock every morning to prepare my baby boy for his day. I'd bathe, clothe, feed, and care for him in general. He adored lavender baths and would oftentimes fall asleep afterwards. He was fond of playing in the bathtub since he loved kicking and splashing the water out of his little blue tub. Getting his hair brushed was heaven on earth for him, and his binky was his everything, He would literally jump out of his bassinet for it.

Big Mama thought I was doing a great job at being a mother, but there was one thing she hated. I was holding Ja'Marcus too much. "You don't want a spoil baby." is what my granny would say often. Since Ja'Marcus was my first child, I was very protective of him like most first-time mothers. I rarely put him in his swing, I did not let him out of my sight, and I absolutely refused to put him on the floor. I was merely afraid he would hurt himself. One summer day, Big Mama was scolding me for holding him. "Get a quilt, spread it out on the floor, and put him down. Right now," Big Mama yelled, so I did.

After putting him on the floor, I was amazed at what I witnessed my son do. At 6 ½ -months-old my child was scooting, crawling, and pulling up. He was all over the house; literally. I remember Big Mama saying "unless you put him down, you will never know what he can do. You can't hold him all the time." I really had no idea he could do the things he was doing. From that point, I continued to put him on the floor every day. Months later he made a major milestone, walking. This was a happy momma moment. My son was growing up.

Ja'Marcus was light skinned, but certain areas of his body were lighter than his actual skin tone. I didn't know what was wrong with him, so I relied on Big Mama for answers. "Get the Vaseline and moisturize his skin" is what she would tell me. Big Mama thought

Vaseline would cure anything. The Vaseline moisturized his skin for a short period, but it did not stop the itch. At times, he would scratch uncontrollably until he would bleed, since his skin was dry. He was always in discomfort, and that made me uncomfortable.

I soon took him to his pediatrician for the skin condition, and learned he had a skin condition known as eczema. The doctor explained eczema is a common condition of the skin where areas of one's skin becomes itchy, inflamed and rough. The medication that was prescribed for him did not ease his distress. There were certain foods he could not eat and beverages that he could not drink. I did not learn this until later. Foods and beverages such as scale fish, chocolate, seafood, oranges, tomato products, milk, egg whites, and plain white bread made the condition worsen. This was a bomber because eggs, chocolate, and orange juice were a few of his favorite foods. He'd been drinking orange juice every day since he was 6 months old. This was the major reason why his skin had become so irritated. Therefore, I had to substitute his favorite juice for apple juice.

I wanted to be a "perfect mother", therefore I would bathe Ja'Marcus 3 times a day. Just to learn I was contributing to his skin being excessively dry. "Too much bathing and staying in water for a long period dries the skin of one with eczema." Dr. Bolt explained. This is the day I found out there is no such thing as being a "perfect mother." I scheduled an appointment for him to see a dermatologist, Dr. Iman. He made one suggestions that will keep Ja'Marcus comfortable. SHOTS! He hated getting shots, and I hated for him get them. I think I would cry more than he would after getting the shot, but the eczema shot every 6 months in his little hip was the only treatment that would stop him from itching. At the end of the day, we both were happy campers. *Eczema is merely a skin condition, my son would surely live.*

"**Momma, you are the best momma in the world! I love you so much. You're my momma and you're my best friend. I can tell you anything. You've been right by my side the entire time. I love you Momma.**"

-Ja'Marcus Davon Davis (2013)

Through the Years
Chapter 3

I went to every prenatal appointment, and I had no complications during my pregnancy. My labor and delivery went well, and we were discharged from the hospital on the third day. Growing up, Ja'Marcus appeared to be a healthy child, despite common childhood illnesses, such as colds, sore throat, fever, and thrush. He was likely to getting ear infections quite frequently, but it was nothing an antibiotic couldn't cure.

Through the years, Ja'Marcus' Head Start, elementary, and middle school years were amazing. He was a gifted child and highly intelligent. He loved going to school and in the second grade he began reading chapter books, since reading was his favorite subject. Ja'Marcus would bring books home from the school's library and read for hours. While in elementary school, he was the only boy in the third grade to win a bike for reading the most books and summarizing them. He loved to talk, and he would get in trouble often at school for it.

Nevertheless, he was an honor student. He was naturally smart, for he rarely studied, yet passed his exams. He loved clothes, and he kept up with the latest fashion. He labeled himself as a trendsetter, for he believed setting trends were cooler than following them.

Ruleville Central Elementary School

"Tigers"

He was diagnosed with Attention Deficit Hyperactivity Disorder or ADHD in elementary school because of his hyperactivity and excessive talking. ADHD is a brain ailment patent by a constant pattern of inattentiveness or hyperactivity impulsiveness that hinders growth or functioning. My son's grades never suffered, but his behavior needed to be managed more while at school. I never believe he had ADHD. He was an only child for 2 years, so I contributed his behavior to him being amongst his peers. I assumed more busy work would do the trick.

Therefore, I asked his teachers to keep him engaged in other activities, so he would not disrupt the class from boredom once he completed his class assignments. This did not work, and he continued to misbehave. My child was not "bad", but his behavior was causing him to be labeled as such, so I elected for medication.

Months after the diagnosis, he took several medications to try to keep him calm during school hours, but the medicines were to no avail. Strattera was one of the many medications that was prescribed for him. After taking it for nearly 3 weeks, it caused him to become mildly depressed. I immediately stopped giving it to him once I noticed his odd behavior per doctor's order. He would come home from school, walk to his room, close the door, and stayed there until the next morning. Some days he would not eat or drink. I questioned him about it, but he could not describe how he felt. "I just do not feel right" would be his response.

I'd tried several medications when I finally decided it was time out for drugs. There were too many negative side effects, besides, none of the medications helped. I talked to a co-worker concerning his condition. She said she was experiencing a similar situation with her foster children.

The way she dealt with them was by keeping them busy with outside activities. "Smart children will act out when they have nothing to do." she said. Indeed, my son was highly intellectual since he passed the gifted test that was administered to him in the 1st grade. Upon hearing this, I did just as she instructed.

Ruleville Middle School

"Bulldogs"

During his 7th grade year at Ruleville Middle School, his last period teacher was very observant. She noticed he began to go to sleep in her class from day-to-day. She originally told me to monitor him at home, but after a week, she became more concerned about him. One afternoon, I was at the school doing my weekly behavior check, she pulled me to the side in the hallway next to her classroom. She told me to take him to the doctor as soon as possible, since she felt something was certainly going wrong with him. For the first time, his grades began to suffer. I was very disturbed by this; therefore, I immediately took him to see a sleep doctor in Greenwood.

The day of the appointment, I was asked several questions concerning his sleep pattern, after which, he was scheduled for a sleep study a few weeks later at Greenwood Leflore Hospital.

Once the sleep study was completed, the nurse informed me he stopped breathing 75 times during the night. He was diagnosed with Sleep Apnea. I was floored! I had no idea my son had a sleep disorder, but with the proper treatment he could live a normal life.

A few weeks later, a tall slender man arrived at our home with Ja'Marcus' C-Pap machine. A C-Pap machine is designed to prevent one's airway from collapsing when he or she breaths in while they are asleep. I was given clear orders on how to put his mask on nightly, how to properly adjust, sanitize, and fill the machine with the adequate amount of water. The device assisted him enormously. He wore his mask faithfully every night and during naps. Ja'Marcus had a mask that he loved, because it was the *perfect* fit. Everything was peaches and cream with his C-Pap machine, until the puppy chewed his favorite mask. He was extremely upset, and his love for the puppy changed.

After receiving his new mask, he was all set. A few weeks later, he was going to school, not falling asleep and he started to bring his grades up. At this point, I knew the C-Pap machine was benefiting him. My job has always been to ensure my son was healthy. Like eczema, this condition did not pose a threat to his life. My son would surly live.

Jay's Hobbies

Ja'Marcus enjoyed drawing, singing, playing video games, football, writing songs, rapping, talking to girls (of course), and playing basketball. This may have been when he discovered he had a great passion for basketball. His favorite basketball player was Brandon Jennings and his favorite team was the L. A. Lakers.

Being a basketball player was his dream, but **cancer** would soon snatch my son's lifelong dream away from him. He played basketball every chance that he had. He liked to play football and he was a huge Michael Vick fan. He and I both were fearful of him getting hurt on the football field, so we both agreed basketball would be the better sport.

He, his brother, and the other children from our small rural town would play basketball every day in the afternoon. Ja'Marcus found a trophy to make their basketball games feel realistic. He practiced day and night since this sport was his life. Basketball was his everything for it appeared to give him life. He played basketball for the Cleveland Park Commission and was awarded 2 consecutive years for participation. Receiving the trophies made him feel as if he'd won a NBA championship.

My son was blessed with many talents. Other than playing basketball, he could sing. I heard Ja'Marcus signing the chorus of Chris Brown's song "Poppin" on jammin' 104 one evening while joyriding. I was mesmerized by his voice. My child could really sing. I sat there quietly and listened. When the song went off, I said to him, "God has blessed you with a beautiful voice. If you can sing R&B, you can sing for Lord." He gave me a long stare, as if he knew where I was going with the conversation, and he did. I was heading straight to the church house. The members of the body always welcomed and encouraged the young members to step up and use their God giving talents. This was Ja'Marcus' chance use what God had blessed him with. Sunday afternoon after worship service, I borrowed a songbook from the church and I started teaching him how to be an effective song leader of the church.

A mother's love for her children has no boundaries.

Church Boy

Chapter 4

Going to church was never an option at our house. I would take out my children's church attire on a Saturday evening to ensure they had no excuses Sunday morning. I did not want Ja'Marcus growing up believing church was a place to sleep. For this reason, he went to bed on Saturday nights as if he was going to school the next day.

During his toddler years, I'd take his miniature toys, crayons, and paper to keep him entertained while Brother Moore preached. Once he reached the age of about 5, I thought it was time for him to learn how one must act during worship. He was now done playing with his favorite little yellow bus, he was now sitting quietly on the pew next to me with his paper, playing as if he was taking notes.

At the age of 8, Ja'Marcus heard and obeyed the Gospel of Christ, and was baptized into the Lord's body. Ja'Marcus could sing like a mockingbird, but he was shy. I did not want to force him to get before the congregation to sing and he became mute. He was around the age of 12 before he became an active song leader. Ja'Marcus was the youngest song leader at Delmar, leading the church in spiritual hymns as if he'd been singing for years. Neither one of us imagined he'd be a song leader, but God works in wonderful ways. To give him a sense of comfort, I told him to look at me if he became nervous. Can you believe Ja'Marcus was a teenage song leader, that was still looking at his momma for comfort while singing? "When the Saints Go Marching In" was his favorite song. He was nothing short of amazing. The congregation encouraged him often, and the churchgoer's kind words were his inspiration since he began leading songs every Sunday.

Annual Youth Conferences

The churches of Christ host an annual Youth Conference. The conference allows youth from different churches of Christ to showcase their talents through speeches and talents. A brother of the church, Kelvin Davis saw Ja'Marcus had the ability to compete in the conference. Ja'Marcus worked hard each year for he was excited to perform for Christ. Therefore, Brother Kevin and his mother Sister Barbara worked faithfully with him on learning and perfecting his speech and talent. They taught him how to bring his talent to the stage and truly use his God-giving abilities. The hard work paid off. He held the title of Mr. Congeniality in 2011 and 2012 for the state of MS and First Runner-Up at National in 2011 and 2012.

It was a privilege and an honor for my son to run in the Youth Conference. The conference is not a place simply to exhibit one's talent, but a place for youth to get closer to Christ and to meet new people. These conferences helped my son to build self-confidence and allowed him to discover new things about himself he was not aware of as well as being able to fearlessly stand before a crowd.

"Train up a child in the way he should go: even when he is old, he will not depart from it."

Proverbs 22:6 (ESV)

Mustard Seed Faith

Ja'Marcus' battle with **cancer** was not a spiritual loss.

For nothing took his eyes off Jesus' glorious cross.

Mustard seed faith was engraved in his heart.

He was rather unique, Christ set him apart.

The faith he exhibited was more than indisputable.

For this walk of life, he was most suitable.

"Have you considered my servant Job?" where the words the Lord uttered to the devil.

Were these words considered for my son, as he prepared for another level?

Cancer was his Goliath and he stood up to fight like David.

I was blessed to have a son, that was specially created.

He fought his giant, and like David, he prevailed.

He left behind a powerful testimony with infinite avail.

He gained the victory through death, though he died not in vain.

His message was designed to equip you, as you will have heartache and pain.

Life will bring storms and for this we must be prepared.

To put on the whole armor of God for the Bible has declared.

You cannot fight without a sword and shield.

You'll need this gear before you get on the battlefield.

Therefore, count it all joy when life's thunderstorm is over your head.

Hebrews 13:5; I will never leave or forsake you; that is what God said.

The book we call the Bible is a book we should all adore.

For Ja'Marcus obeyed The Gospel and this Lucifer could not destroy.

Babes in Christ are fragile, they are easy to bend and break.

They need more understanding, more storms of life before entering the pearly gates.

Ja'Marcus was grounded in the word of God as he had what it took.

For mature men of God feast on strong meat and their faith is trained by The Book. Revelation 14:13 gave my son unwavering peace and joy.He put away childish things, for he was not a boy.

A crown of righteousness, he was prepared to wear.

When my number is called, I hope to meet him there.

His Gut Instinct

Chapter 5

Ja'Marcus was attending Ruleville Central High School when he began to complain of stomach pain. He went to school one morning slightly hurting, but the pain was tolerable. As the day continued the pain became unbearable, therefore, he put his head on the desk. I am an extremely firm parent, and I believe in my children going to school doing what he or she is supposed to do with no disrespect. Coach JJ knew this, and he would text me every other day concerning Ja'Marcus' "disrespectful" behavior. I made it my business to go to the school to discuss the matter because Ja'Marcus was not being raised to be bad-mannered.

After getting off work, I walked to the school. Before I walked through the door, I said a quick prayer in order that I might remain humble. I saw Coach JJ in the hallway, and he hurriedly walked to me as if he knew I was there to see him. He smiled and excitedly pulled out his cell phone. We greeted each other, and he immediately showed me a video that he had recorded earlier of the encounter he had with Ja'Marcus. I watched the video closely without saying a word. I listened to every word that was spoken. He walked to my son's desk and asked him to hold his head up and complete his assignment. Appearing to be in pain, Ja'Marcus tells him, "I am doing my work Coach. My head is down because my stomach is hurting." He proceeded to tell my son, "I know your mother wants what is best for you, but I don't see you passing my class, not this year." Ja'Marcus did not respond neither did he raise his head up from the desk. He stood by Jay's desk for a while, then he soon walked away.

After watching the video, I brought to his attention the statement when my son said he was not feeling well and the statement he made concerning him not passing his class. At this point, I had to walk down the hallway a pray again, because he was pushing all the wrong buttons. He was unbelievably nonchalant as an educator and inconsiderable as a human. My son's pain was not a concern him, but the class assignment was. I was furious since my son admired this coach to the fullest. How could he be so heartless? My son, his student was in excruciating pain, and his primary concern was for him to hold his head up, and complete his work. To me it did not matter if his head was up or down, as long as he was completing the assignment. With that initial conversation, my mind was made up. I'd had enough of him and Ruleville Central High School.

My son's journey as a Tiger was over! The next morning, Ja'Marcus stayed home with Big Mama while I went to RCHS to withdraw him.

A New Beginning

"Trojans Never Say Die in the Face of Defeat"

The next week, I enrolled him at East Side High School in Cleveland, MS. I initially wanted him to attend Cleveland High School, but we were not in the Cleveland High School zone, and for that reason he had to attend East Side High. Ja'Marcus' first day at East Side High did not go as he planned. When I inquired about his first day, he without delay said, "it did not go well Momma. I do not like it! I really want to go to Cleveland High." We discussed what happened, and why he could not attend CHS. We prayed that day two would be better, and it was.

When I made it home from work the next afternoon, he was lying down. I peeped my head inside his room, and asked "how was your day today?" "I loved it! I know everyone there." he told me. "This is the best class at East Side. Class of 2014" he excitingly said. I was happy because he was happy and content. I was grateful day two was better, because sending him back to Ruleville Central High School was out of the equation. East Side High School was everything I hoped it would be for my son. He loved the staff, especially the counselor Mrs. Holmes. She was the heart of the school in Ja'Marcus' eyes. Every day, he had something positive to say about her. I was never called to the school for his conduct or grades. He took a course at the Vocational Center. Talking has always been Ja'Marcus' biggest problem in school. I received 2 certified letters in the mail from his Votex teachers concerning his behavior on two different occasions. Talking and swearing he had "swag" (as the young generation says) is what always got him in trouble.

He would ask to go to the bathroom, but instead of him going back to class and taking his seat, he would stand for minutes fixing his clothes. After being told several times to sit down, he failed to cooperate and for this reason, he was written up. The Cleveland School District during this time would send out certified letters to parents for their child's misconduct. The teachers would know the letter was received since an adult had to sign for it. We all know that children will tell what everyone else does at school, but they'll never tell on themselves. For this reason, I was thankful for Cleveland School District because I like to stay knowledgeable on what my child is doing while at school. I expected for him and his siblings to go to school and behave and if they were disobedient; there are consequences. Ja'Marcus' cell phone was his second heartbeat.

After he lost his cell phone privileges, he quickly learned I was not tolerating negative behavior. Over the next months, his teacher began to see a positive change in him, and he was voted as Mr. FCCLA (Family, Career and Community Leaders of America). He was excited about representing East Side and Cleveland High School, and he did so with honor, pride and dignity.

I would make it home daily after 6 because I would stop by Big Mama's house to check on her. Every day that I made it home, Ja'Marcus would be asleep. He would eat cereal and leave the bowl and spoon in the sink every day. I would wash the dishes, until one day I said, "It is only a bowl and spoon Ja'Marcus. Why don't you wash it?" "Every day I come home Momma, my stomach hurts after I eat. I put the dishes in the sink and lay down because I planned on washing it later." were his words. Now, being the mother that I am; I was not buying that same excuse every day. I said to him, "every day that you come home, you're able to eat with no problem, but when it is time to wash the dishes, your stomach hurt?" "Yes ma'am. I know it doesn't sound right, but I am telling the truth." He went on to point out where the pain was coming from. Since the pain was on and off, I did not believe it to be too serious. Our conversations did not change anything. He would still come home, eat, put the dishes in the sink, and go to bed.

After a few weeks, he complained about stomach pain constantly, but he could attend school daily.

East Side High School's motto was ***"Trojans never say die in the face of defeat"***, and this motto fully described my son. He was a true TROJAN! He pushed through pain every day, because he wanted to live a normal life. He assured me he was fine, but it wasn't until later I learned he was in more pain than he claimed.

He and I were in the living room one afternoon conversing, when he stood up and asked, "Momma, where is your liver?" I did not want anything to be wrong with my him, so I was sarcastic when I said, "Google it. You Google everything else." He believed the pain that he was experiencing was coming from his liver. I told him that I would take him to the doctor to get an order to have a liver test done, because he was previously on medication for ADHD. When one takes medication for ADHD, he or she must have their liver checked periodically. We laughed off my "Google it" statement and he went outside to play basketball.

The next day, I took him to the doctor as a walk-in patient. I told the doctor what needed to be done, he complied with no hesitancy, and wrote the order. My son and I walked to Bolivar Medical Center to get the test done. I prayed and patiently waited for the results. After a week, the tests results came back, and they were "negative." Everything was "fine" according this test. I was pleased to tell him the news. He was glad to hear the results, but he still felt in his soul that something was wrong with his liver. Four months later, his ***gut instinct*** would be accurate.

Lord my God, I called you for help, and you healed me.

Psalm 30:2 (NIV)

A Ray of Hope
Chapter 6

During Spring Break of 2013, Ja'Marcus and his siblings were in Ruleville with our grandmother and aunts. I was at home asleep when my Aunt Margaret called me around 11:20 pm to tell me that Ja'Marcus was in excruciating pain. I quickly put on a pair of jeans and a t-shirt. I rushed to tell my husband I was heading to Ruleville to take Ja'Marcus to the clinic. I grabbed my keys and gym shoes and rushed out the door. As I drove 85 mph down the highway, I prayed to God there were no state troopers out. My son needed to see a doctor, therefore stopping was not in the plan.

Who would have imagined, we would make 4 consecutive ER and clinic visits before my son had a diagnosis?

Visit 1~Wednesday

Thank God, the clinic closed at 12:00 a.m. and no one was there. I signed in at 11:35 and shortly after arriving my son's round black beeper started to light up. It was time to see the doctor.

After my son's vitals were taken, we were escorted to a room halfway down the hall. Ja'Marcus was holding his stomach indicating he was in serious pain and he was constantly vomiting. We walked into room number seven, and Ja'Marcus walked directly to the examination table and laid down. After being asked several questions concerning the reason for the visit, blood was drawn, and his blood pressure was taken. His pressure was good, and the blood work came back 25 minutes later normal. He was not giving any medication for pain or vomiting, since there was a stomach bug going around during the time. The ER physician "presumed" he had come across a germ. He was diagnosed with a stomach virus. Before leaving the ER, his pain had subsided to about a level four and the vomiting ceased

I wanted to take him home with me, so I could keep a watchful eye on him. He convinced me that he felt better, and to let him stay at Big Mama's house. While getting out of the truck, I questioned him carefully about his pain, and he said, "I am good Momma. I promise."

I did not want to over react. I agreed to let him stay, and I walked him in the house. I updated my aunt on the possible diagnosis. Before leaving, I told her to call me without delay if he needed me, and shortly after I headed home.

Visit 2~Thursday

At 9:00 AM my phone rang. It was my aunt. "Ja'Marcus need to see a doctor right away, because he is hurting really bad'', is what she yelled. I was still dressed from the previous ER visit. I put on my gym shoes, grabbed my keys and headed out the door...again.

During this visit, I quickly informed the triage nurse that we were just at the ER. Blood work had been done and it came back normal and he was diagnosed with a stomach bug. If I told you that the entire health professional team seemed to be as perplexed as I was, would you believe me? That is exactly how they appeared. They were standing there acting and looking confused. I had to tell them what test to run because I doubt if he had a stomach virus. "Give him an X-ray because something is going on with his stomach" is what I angrily uttered. They all instantly agreed and nearly 15 minutes later, an X-ray technician came, took him to the back, and completed the X-Ray. A doctor later came in and told me the x-ray determined he was compacted. I was greatly relieved because now I have an answer to why he is in severe pain (at least that's what I thought). He was written a prescription for a laxative. This will fix the problem. The prescription for the Miralax was filled at the local pharmacist, and once again we were on our way home.

Now surly if I give him the laxative, he would be fine. Boy, was I wrong! By the time, we arrived home, he was vomiting severely. I could not give him the medication because there was no way it was going to stay down. He could not eat or drink. Later in the evening, the vomiting subsided, and he could tolerate a cup of juice and Miralax. He was successful. He did not vomit, and the laxative did what it was supposed to do (several times). I was thankful, and assumed he was merely constipated...until later that night.

Ja'Marcus was computer savvy. He decided to Google "stabbing stomach pain", and appendicitis mimicked his symptoms. He carefully read the article, and it read "sitting in a tub of warm water would ease the appendicitis pain. He told my aunt about what he'd read, and she ran him some bath water to sit in, eagerly praying this would ease his pain, and it did. Once he got out of the tub the pain returned before long. I figured that holding a warm towel would ease the pain just as sitting in the warm water would. I was right, but once the warm packs started to cool, the pain would come back unbearable. We continued to hold warm compresses on his abdomen the rest of the night for relief.

I was feed up with the doctors because despite the x-ray results, I felt in my heart that something was seriously wrong with my son. I was no longer mad, I was furious. I had to push them to run test on Jay to determine why he was in grave pain. It was not my job to tell them what to do. I am not a medical professional. On the other hand, a mother must do what a mother must do. I was not going to sit quietly while they did nothing, and I was not going to stop until I knew why my child was in such discomfort.

Visit 3~Friday

Three days had passed, and my son was still in constant agony

. Today was not the day! I was not in the mood for a game of cat and mouse with the doctors. I was going to get some answers concerning my son's health. I was not going to stop until I had a clear diagnosis.

I signed in and waited until Ja'Marcus Davis' name was called. After being at the clinic 3 days in a row, there was no need for us to go triage. The health professional knew what was going on by now. We were called to an examination room, where the on-call doctor looked over my son's file from the previous visits. My patients were short, and before he could finish reading, I said "I have given him the laxative, and he has been to be bathroom several times. Now can I have another x-ray to see if he is still compacted." The doctor agreed, and minutes later the x-ray technician came with a wheelchair and took him to the x-ray lab. The x-ray tech clearly explained what she was doing and after 4 pictures of Jay's abdomen had been taken, a doctor would later come and read the results.

"Everything looks good" is what the doctor told me. I was not buying that today. "No, everything may look good, but it is not good. I need further test ran" is what I harshly stated. "Could the pain he's having be appendicitis?" I asked as calmly as possible. "No, his appendix looks fine." he stated. "Well how about a sonogram of his belly and a MRI" were my next words. I was absolutely bewildered at the fact that I had to make suggestions on what to do next.

I shook my head in disbelief and impatiently waited on the doctor's response. It only took him a few seconds to agree with me, but it felt like hours. The MRI was done at the hospital immediately. The sonogram was scheduled for the following Monday. Monday was just 4 days away, but the wait seemed forever.

We sat calmly waiting on the MRI to be done. Then walks a short, funny, and happy-go-lucky man. I was so glad to see someone that was upbeat because he quickly managed to put a smile on Ja'Marcus and my face. He walked in stepping high and full of joy, but with a sincere sense of caring in his heart.

"Let's get this young man ready for the MRI" is what he stated, while looking me eye to eye. He asked me question after question concerning Jay and his health. It's odd because he asked more questions than the doctors asked. At this moment, I felt as if I was going to get some answers.

Ja'Marcus was in pain as the radiologist technician prepped him and assisted him as he sat on the scanner for the MRI. I walked in the room with him close to where Jay was located. He closed the door, pressed a small button and asked Ja'Marcus if he was ok before he started the MRI. "Yes sir" was Jay's reply. When he was in pain, he did not want to or like to talk, so I can imagine how he felt. The X-ray technician held me a casual conversation for a few minutes, and then suddenly he became awfully quiet; too quiet. The room was so calm I became instantly nervous.

Then from out the blue, he said, "Do you see this?" as he moved the computer's mouse over the spot. "Yes, I see it", I anxiously said aloud. "Well, this is fluid and it is not supposed to be in his belly" he said. He continued to shake his head as if he was in disbelief and looked at the computer screen. He maneuvered the mouse around faster and faster, and that was my indication that something was utterly wrong, but I had no idea it was as critical as it was.

"I'll let the doctor look at these scans, and he will let you know what he will do from here" is what the X-ray tech sadly said. He was no longer smiling and to have appeared to be crying. Ja'Marcus and I went back to the rural clinic to wait for the results, when a nurse came and told me that they would call me with the results.

Later that afternoon, my phone rang. I looked at the number, and initially started not to answer, because I normally do not answer calls I don't recognize. After the 3rd ring, I quickly thought "the clinic" and I answered the call. It was indeed the doctor. My heart was beating uncontrollably as I walked outside to talk in private. My aunt as concerned, and she followed me out since she noticed my facial expression and tone of voice. My voice trembled like a magnitude 8 earthquake, as I answered the phone. "Hello." I said slowly. "Is this Tawanda." the doctor asked swiftly. "Yes, this is she" I answered. "This is Dr. Hayfield. I am calling concerning your son's test results. The MRI showed spots on your son's liver. This does not mean that he has **cancer**. We do need to run additional test. He has an appointment for a sonogram at the Sunflower Diagnostic Center on Monday at 9:30 a.m." the doctor said. The only word that could come out of my mouth was "okay." "Be sure to take him and be there on time" he added. I frantically hung up the phone without a goodbye. Job 17:15(NIV) instantly came to my mind: where then is my hope-who can see any hope for me. At that very moment, all I had was a ***ray of hope***.

Yet there is one ray of hope. His compassion never ends. It is only the Lord's mercies that have kept us from complete destruction.

Lamentations 3:21-22 (TLB)

Lord Why?

Chapter 7

I looked to the heavens with heart wrenching pain. I knew even at my lowest point God was watching over me. In a soft tone, I spoke, "**Lord why**?" "What have I done wrong?" "What if my child has **cancer**?" "What am I supposed to do?" "What is he supposed to do?" "What has he done to deserve this?" are the questions I uttered to God over and over. I felt as if I was having an outer body experience. This could not be true. I was trying like crazy to wrap my mind around the words the doctor told me the previous day. I did not want to believe it was **cancer**, because spots do not mean **cancer**. I did not want to picture the fact that my son may die at such a young age, but the thought kept playing over and over in my head.

My thoughts were racing like the Indy 500, that my mind could hardly keep up. My heart suddenly rewinds back to earlier months before Ja'Marcus became ill. I had taken him to the doctor for a routine check-up. The nurse practitioner had nearly completed the check-up, when he decided to check his lymph nodes.

After checking them he made the statement the lymph nodes were swollen. He also said that swollen lymph nodes were a sign of **cancer.** Hearing the word **cancer** has always alarmed me. This 6-letter word is so small, but it is enormously powerful. I refused to listen to anything else the he had to say. I immediately got my son and left the clinic; only hearing the doctor say, "bring him back in a few days so I can check his lymph nodes again." After three days, I took him back to the doctor and surprisingly his lymph nodes were no longer swollen. Since they had decrease in size, **cancer** was no longer an option; I THOUGHT!

Can I just be honest for a minute? When the doctor said the word "spots", the first thing that came to mind was **cancer**. If we all would be honest, **cancer** would be your primary thoughts as well. Just hearing the word **cancer** makes most people overwhelmed, hysterical, and numb. I felt in my spirit my faith was being tested once again. I will pass the test, and God will get the glory.

Visit 4~ Monday

Today is the day of truth. We will learn my son's fate. I had a major pity party in my grandmother's lawn the day before, but faith was all I had to embrace. I prayed. I begged God to make a way for us to have peace. He hadn't brought us this far to leave. Whatever the diagnosis maybe, God was still in control. Surely God is my help; the Lord is the one who sustains me. Psalms 54:4 (NIV) is one of the many scriptures that I mediated on while I waited for answers.

I entrusted my son in the hands of my husband and aunt. They would take care of him and have him at his appointment on time. I was sitting at the table with my Kindergarten students, when my mind begins to roam with thoughts. "It is **cancer**. Your son has **cancer**" are the thoughts that raced through my mind as I passed out the children's morning assignment. I could not get the idea out of my mind. Once the sonogram was completed, my aunt texted me. "The doctor will call you with the results." Is what it read.

I received a phone call from the clinic while I was at work relating to my son, but I did not take the call. I did not want to hear any bad news while I was at work. I immediately told my supervisor what was going on, and I left work. I stopped by the house first to pick up my son and husband, and we headed to the rural clinic. We did not have to sign in since the doctors were awaiting our arrival. One of the two doctors escorted us to an examination room, while the other doctor went to his office. We sat in the room and readily waited for the test results. No one looked as if they were nervous, but we were. The negative feeling of my son having **cancer** were no longer a factor in my heart. After waiting for nearly an hour, I became extremely anxious and impatient.

Later, the doctor that accompanied us to the examination room knocked on the door. "Come in" I replied. He pointed to me and asked me to follow him. He was walking a mile a minute. I could barely keep up since I felt in me spirt that something was unbearably wrong, but I prayed my initial thoughts about **cancer** were not right. I followed the doctor to a small room, there he gave me a large yellow folder, and with an oddly loud voice stated, "you wanted to know what was wrong with your son, right? "Yes, I do" I answered with a hopeful tone. "He has **cancer**. The MRI and sonogram showed spots on your son's liver. I have already scheduled him an appointment in Jackson, MS at Blair E. Batson Children's Hospital. It looks very bad. I set his appointment up for this Thursday." I was taken back. I stood there in absolute disbelief with complete silence and a blank stare on my face. I was struck with complete shock with undefined horror and in absolute awe! The doctor was very careless with his words and extremely unsympathetic concerning my feelings as a mother. I was overwhelmed and saddened.

Did I hear this man correctly? Did he just say the word that no one man or woman wants to hear? **CANCER**! Did he really say to me my son had **cancer**? These thoughts rushed through my brain at 100 miles per hour. I looked at him one last time thinking, "This was a mistake. They have assuredly gotten my son's file confused with someone else's."

They looked at me and said no more. I took a deep breath as a grasped the envelope. I swallowed and slowly tried to find my way back to the room where my son and husband were waiting. Now what? How could I tell my son that he had been diagnosed with **cancer**?

After hearing the results, one word came to my mind "DEATH." "My son was going to leave me." My son was going to die? How am I supposed to live without my firstborn? Lord, why have you chosen me to fight this battle and why did you choose my child? These were the words that I expressed out aloud on the way home with great resentment towards God. My faith was being tested for a third time, but this time was going to be different than the other two times. I was determined to pass the test, but I wanted answers. I needed answers. Jesus had the answers, and I wanted to know. How could He give me my first child, and possibly take him away? I've dealt with eczema, ADHD, and sleep apnea, but **cancer** was a new level. Will my son die? I'll hold God's hand, and I will learn our fate. **Cancer** is limited, it will not destroy my son's faith.

and said: "Naked I came from my mother's womb, and naked I will depart. The Lord gave and the Lord has taken away; may the name of the Lord be praised."

-Job 1:21(NIV)

Sharing the News

Chapter 8

No one can imagine how I felt as I walked back to the examination room. I thought my heart was going to beat out of my chest. With every step, it seemed to beat faster. These palpations lasted for nearly an hour. Scared was an understatement. I was in absolute fear.

I am terrible with directions. Finding the room where Ja'Marcus and Jermaine were waiting took me forever. After looking in 5 empty rooms, I finally made it. I weakly pushed the door open and said, "Let's go!" I was trying to hold my composure and not faint at the same time.

"What did they say?" Jermaine asked. I was not in the mood to talk, so I said quickly "I'll tell you when we get home." "What did the doctor say Momma?" my son eagerly asked looking perplexed. I was completely speechless for nearly 2 minutes. I gazed into his small brown eyes and tried to figure out exactly what to say and how to say it. I was speechless. I wanted to talk, but nothing would come out of my mouth. Ja'Marcus loudly asked again, "Momma, what is it? What is wrong with me?" I was so hurt, I angrily uttered, "Do you really want to know what is wrong with you Ja'Marcus?" "Yes ma'am. I do." he said looking down. "You have **cancer** Son. The doctor said you have **cancer**." By this time, tears flowed down my cheek bones. Ja'Marcus and my husband were mute, and the room was silent. Ja'Marcus dropped his head and put his arms around my waist. My emotions were crazy. I soon gathered my composure, and we slowly walked out of clinic in silence. As we were walking to the truck, I walked alongside my son for consolation., for he was now sobbing. I sat with him during the ride home, for comfort.

    We pulled in the driveway hoping that this was all a dream. "Do you want me to tell the kids?" I asked him. "No ma'am. I will tell them." he said with a low tone. He opened the door of the truck, and we sluggishly walked in the house. I had called my Aunt Margaret and cousin Ann while we were in route home and told them the devastating news. They could not believe their ears. I dreaded to tell my cousin, because her mother had been diagnosed with lung **cancer** and she already dealing with a lot. I informed her on our next step. Shortly after our brief conversation, we prayed one for another, and ended our disheartening talk. As we were getting out of the vehicle, Ja'Marcus spoke these words without a tear in sight, "I knew something was wrong with me, but I didn't know it was **cancer**. I am going to pray about it and start eating healthy. I will fine."

We walked in the house hand in hand.

Jermaine went to pick the kids up from school, and around 4:00 they arrived home. They spoke to Big Mama and walked into the living room where everyone was sitting. Someone asked, "What's wrong? Why are you all sitting in here?" I could not speak, because I still trying to wake up from this nightmare. Sitting in the living room wasn't normal for us, so they knew something wasn't quite right. "Go and put your bookbags up.

"I have something to tell you." Ja'Marcus told them. I had never seen my children look as confused as they were now. Maybe they felt the thick tension coming from us. At once, they hurried back into the living room, sat down, and looked at me. I knew **sharing the news** wasn't going to be an easy task, therefore, I wanted to tell the children myself, but I felt it would be better if they heard it from Ja'Marcus. Minutes passed without anyone saying a word. Ja'Marcus and I looked at each other with a faint smile, and he spoke these words; "I have **cancer**." It was like a bomb had dropped right in our living room. Eyes bucked, mouths dropped, and tears fell. There was not a dry eye in the house, expect Ja'Marcus' eyes. My children were in excruciating pain from hearing this overwhelming news. He had already started displaying his faith. Then suddenly he said; "Don't cry for me. I am going to be fine. I am going to the hospital Thursday. I'll be back home soon" he said in an upbeat voice. His words of comfort did not stop the tears.

Ja'Marcus and his siblings were very close. I understood this was going to take a toll on them, for this reason; I had to be strong.

I needed prayers and spiritual comfort, so I contacted my minister and his wife. Brother Billy and Sister Deborah Moore were there from the beginning. With just one phone call, they were knocking at the door. God was with me, but I needed people. Only God could bring me out, but prayers would certainly help me. This was a storm that I did not have to fight alone, and I was thankful I didn't have too. We needed spiritual guidance now more than ever. I told them what the doctors told me, and immediately we went to God in prayer.

Around 7:30 that evening, I went to Facebook to vent. A sister from the church, who is a nurse practitioner saw the status I had posted, and she immediately contacted Sister Flowers who is also a nurse practitioner to check on us since she would get off work before she did. God is good! Sister Flowers came to the house to check on us immediately after work. I was glad to see her because I needed someone to explain to me what the doctors did not. She walked to my son's room, raised his shirt up, and looked at his fluid filled and swollen abdomen. Having fluid in the abdomen is medically known as ascites, she explained to me. I told her what the doctors told me and I gave her the envelope of papers, sonogram images and MRI scans. The doctors had diagnosed my son with a form of **cancer**, but he did not tell me what kind of **cancer**.

Sister Flowers felt he should not have told me Ja'Marcus had **cancer**, because a biopsy had not been performed to determine it that were true. "A biopsy is a sample of tissue taken from the body to examine it more closely." she explained. Every question I asked, she answered it in everyday terms. She was more than helpful to my son and I. Doctors use medical terms that are long and sometimes hard to pronounce. Sister Flowers clarified all the medical terms to me where I could better understand. Her being there meant so much to my son and me.

Even though we knew we were not alone, sometimes it felt as if we were. At times, we feel that we can walk this earth without people and that is not true. There will come a time in life when you will need somebody's help. This world is too big to not need help at some point and time. Therefore, we should love and treat everyone the way we want to be treated for we never know who hands will fall in.

Ja'Marcus got out the bed for a while, after Sister Flowers left. He was not in pain, and that was a blessing. His siblings were still greatly concerned about him. The boys went in the room with him to keep him company until he was ready to go back to bed. They talked and laughed half of the night. They really needed this alone time together because we did not know when we were coming back home. I thought Jay would have been down after hearing he had **cancer**, but instead he wasn't. He was in good spirit. Seeing him in a good mood made me happy. When my children are happy, I am happy.

Tawanda L. Davis-Hudson

Do not let your hearts be troubled. You believe in God; believe also in me.

-John 14:1 (NIV)

Preparing for the Storm
Chapter 9

As we prepared for the journey to Blair E. Batson Children's Hospital in Jackson, MS; I was filled with doubts, what ifs, anger, and fear as we were **preparing for the storm**. There were no words that could describe how I felt, but we were blessed to have a God fearing and praying church family. During this time, I learned that God will place certain individuals in your life to help you through your storm. Ja'Marcus had been diagnosed with **cancer** during the same time as our Aunt Shirley's diagnosis. I believe that God allowed her to be in her storm because He knew we were going into the same storm, and we needed the encouragement on our journey from someone that we greatly admired.

Aunt Shirley was such a strong woman of faith. She refused to let **cancer** shun her of her faith which was greater than the size of a mustard seed. She did not let **cancer** keep her from shining bright like the diamond that she was, and she continued to dazzle all that knew her with her cheerful smile. She inspired the both of us from the beginning of the battle.

Aunt Shirley loved shopping and wearing her 3 and 4-inch heels. She did not mind cooking from sun up to sun down for cooking was her passion. There were times I wondered, where did all her strength come from? Then it hit me, she's a praying and God-fearing woman. Proverbs 31:30 (NIV) says, charm is deceptive, and beauty is fleeting; but a woman who fears the Lord is to be praised. This scripture described my aunt perfectly. She prayed about everything and she did not allow the cares of the world to worry her. "Worry? For what?" were he sarcastic, but serious words.

Everything that I mentioned about my Aunt was her and more, but she had one trait that was pure genuine; LOVE. I Peter 4:8 teaches us that love covers a multitude of sins. Her love for people shined like the morning star. It was real and people loved her. Most of all Aunt Shirley loved God and her Delmar Avenue Church of Christ family. Her faith was nothing short of amazing. There was one thing you would not hear my aunt do, and that was complain. "What I'm I complaining about? It will not help." is what she would say. Instead she put her trust in The Highest God and prayed. Her positive outlook on life is just what we needed to fight this battle.

Aunt Shirley and Sister Flowers were such a blessing because they were our backbone. I needed these women like I needed oxygen. I could not have made it without them. I recall telling them "I need both of you to come with us to Jackson.

I do not know what to ask the doctors and I am scared. I am used to asking minor questions about ear infections, colds, eczema, and chickenpox. **cancer** was out of my league, and with Sister Flowers being in the medical field was exactly who we needed. She is incredibly knowledgeable. I was panic-stricken with grief when I found out my son was sick, but she eased my fears with her presence alone.

We gave our final hugs and kisses and said our goodbyes. We did not know how long we would be apart, so I allowed the children to stay home from school, to see us off. It broke my heart to pieces because I had never been away from my children. Everyone was gathered outside chatting before we left, but Ja'Marcus was still in the house in his bedroom. I thought he was getting nervous as the time neared for us to depart. I went back in the house to ensure that he was fine. After talking with him, I was wrong. I was the only one nervous. He was focused on his little brother. He was trying to make sure that he would be okay while he was away. He was indeed a big brother looking out for his younger brother.

Ja'Marcus was the eldest of 9 children. He was exceedingly protective of his siblings. He had a major concern for his younger brother Quoindedrick, whom nickname is Chinney. Chinney is 2 years younger than Jay. In his younger days, he was easily influenced and in my opinion; he made friends with no trouble. I did not like that since sometimes the children that he befriended were not heading down the right path. Chinney had just started his Freshman year at East Side High School when Jay became ill. Ja'Marcus did not want him to attend school in Cleveland because he would not be at school with him, he was small in stature and he had grave concerns of him being bullied. I did not want to upset him, so I assured him that I would withdraw Chinney the following week and enroll him at Ruleville Central High School. Moments later Ja'Marcus approached me in the hallway and stated "Momma, it is okay. Chinney can go to East Side. I have someone looking out for him." I smiled and said, "ok." He had a sense of calmness writing all over his. Even during his time of illness, he was still watching out for his little brother. He was emotionally preparing Chinney for something greater. Later in the story you'll better understand why. Chinney would soon wear the title "big brother."

Knowing that I was heading to a hospital that catered to children, was a major relief. They would surly run the test that were needed, perform the biopsy, treat my son, and we'd be on our way home in no time. My mind began to race with thoughts. It is 2013. Technology has advanced more now than ever. Surly there would be a cure for his **cancer** if it was **cancer**. Therefore, with prayer and a countless number of trained health professionals, there was no doubt that my son was not going to be fine. Clearly since the pain had just started (I thought) the **cancer** is certainly in Stage I. My son was going to kick **cancer's** butt.

During the entire ride to Jackson, no one talked about the possible diagnosis. Before we got in the truck Ja'Marcus prayed, although he was terribly uncomfortable given that he had been vomiting and was in horrific pain. I had purchased a small bottle of nausea medication a few days prior to give to him, but I never opened it. He began to get nauseous from the smell of specific odors, so I did not want to take the chance on making him feel worst. Ja'Marcus began to vomit so bad, I thought he would never stop. Thank God, I had packed plenty of bags, towels, and baby wipes because we certainly needed them.

Normally driving 2 hours to Jackson seems like forever, but not this time. We came in our vehicle, since Aunt Shirley and Sister Flowers were going back home after Ja'Marcus was admitted. We walked inside the hospital, and immediately I became light headed and nauseous. I was so nervous I thought I was going to pass out because I did not know what to expect. Ja'Marcus on the other hand seemed to be fearless.

Once we made it to the hospital, the vomiting subsided for a while chatted. We sat in the lobby of the hospital waiting for Sister Flowers and my aunt to come in. While waiting for them, I walked to the admission desk, checked Jay in and handed the receptionist the envelope that contained Jay's medical documents. Minutes later theycame in and joined us. My Aunt Shirly prayed, and told us that whatever the doctors say, we must hold on to faith.

A female doctor walked out of her office, introduced herself, and asked us to follow her. We walked down the long hallway, and with each step I wanted to turn around and run. I was scared out of my mind. It felt as if I was walking through a haunted house given that my heart was filled with anxiety and uncertainty. This was not my son's primary doctor, even though I prayed it would be. She was an amazing doctor. She was very detailed in explaining what would be taken place over the next few days.

Minutes after she walked in, I Googled her on Healthgrades.com, and she'd scored an A. Sister Flowers had already schooled me a few days earlier about this website. "Always check their grade." is what she uttered in Jay's bedroom, and I did just that.

At this point I was lost, therefore Sister Flowers asked all the questions. The doctor gave clear and direct answers. I would not be able to remember everything that was being said, so I pulled out a pen and a piece of paper from my purse and started taking notes. I had to be knowledgeable of what would be going on with my child. Sister Flowers was helpful, but her physical presence was temporary.

The doctor left the room to ensure that Ja'Marcus' room was prepared. We walked back to the lobby and conversed about what the doctor had discussed with us. Sister Flowers made sure I understood everything before they headed home. I assured her I was ready for the fight. As the doctor was coming to get us, we were saying our final goodbyes. I did not want them to leave, but I knew I had to do this. This is our first journey in the mist of the storm, yet we were not alone. God was with us.

Be strong and courageous. Do not be afraid or terrified because of them, for the LORD your God goes with you; he will never leave you or forsake you.

–Deuteronomy 31:6 (NIV)

Ye of Little Faith
Chapter 10

I believe God always allows one to go through trials and tribulations for a reason. Majority of the time we do not understand why we are in a storm. It is not until the storm is over, we can begin to try to piece together the fragments of life that were destroyed. It is not always simple. Truthfully, it is hard. Life can throw fiery missiles that we never saw coming. The unknown is always frightening, especially when your level of faith is zero. We tend to put on a show for the world, when it comes to Christianity. God sees all, thus, fronting for the world is not needed. Man, cannot condemn us to hell or give us a crown of righteousness. Revelation 3:16 explains that one must be either hot or cold, there is no in between. There is no such thing as lukewarm Christian.

Nevertheless, I played church. I would go to worship service and Bible study when I wanted to. I was not fully dedicated to Him like He was to me. God had shown His mercy and grace towards me just by blessing me with life, but I held up a rebellious fist in His face. I knew Hebrew 10:25 says, "not forsaking the assembling of ourselves together as the manner of some is; but exhorting one another; and so much the more, as ye see the day approaching." I completely ignored the word of God. I knew I was wrong, but I continued to do what pleased me. Playing church caused me to hurt like no other. I did not have on the full armor of God. I was not equipped to fight. Although I recognized what the word of God said, I never studied and meditated on His word. I would soon be at sea and feel alone. Yes, God is there, but I will drown in shallow thoughts of doubts and why me. I didn't understand why God choose me, but He did. He was preparing me for a greater storm.

I went into labor with child number seven on December 2, 2005, but he wasn't due until December 21. I woke up around 6 o'clock AM feeling decreased movement. I wasn't alarmed since babies do not move constantly. I felt extremely tired, so I stayed in the bed until 1 o'clock PM. I finally got up, and went to the bathroom because I felt cramp-like symptoms. I slowly walked back down the hall and into the den with Big Mama. I pulled up a chair beside her, and explained to her how I felt. I was beyond anxious, so I could not sit down. I fell to my knees in pain. Big Mama helped me up, and I proceeded to the bathroom. I heard Big Mama open the door for my Aunt Margaret, and tell her I was sick. I wanted to call her name, but I was in grave pain. She quickly greeted Big Mama, and hurried to me. Neither one of us was ready for what happened next. I started to bleed. I was terrified. She pulled out her cell phone and dialed 911.

After nearly 10 minutes of impatiently waiting and hysterical crying, the paramedics finally arrived. I was transported to Bolivar Medical Center for treatment. After I was rushed to the second floor to an examination room, several registered nurses and certified nurse assistants filled the small room. The nurse grabbed the Aquasonic 100 ultrasound gel and applied a generous amount to my belly, while getting her Doppler.

She moved the Doppler across my belly where she believed she would hear my son's heartbeat. After about 2 minutes of trying to detect a heartbeat, she put the Doppler down and wiped my belly clean. The room was quiet and a few nurses swiftly walked out. "What is wrong?" I screamed. She dropped her head, and replied, "The doctor will be in shortly." Just like her, I heard no heartbeat. I did not need a doctor to tell me what I already assumed. I knew that my baby boy was dead. I wept silently and waited for the doctor's confirmation.

Minutes later, the on-call doctor walked into the room. He with great composure told me my son had passed away due to complete placental abruption. He went on to explain that placental abruption occurs when the placenta separates from the mother's uterus before the baby is born. This deprives the baby of oxygen and nutrients, ending in death. I was given the drug Pitocin to help speed up my labor, and at 5:20 PM, I delivered a 5-pound lifeless baby boy; whom I named Jay'Coreyon Everett (Baby Jay). I was heartbroken.

It was clear that the Lord was punishing me. I failed to do His will, and now I was facing the consequences of His anger. My son was dead, and so was my faith.

I have encountered many tribulations in my life, but I feel there is no greater tribulation than losing a child. "I am a Christian, but at that point, my faith was not mustard seed size." I thought to myself. This is the first time my faith had been tested to this degree. I failed the test. I was so angry with God. "I was not going to church faithfully before I lost my child, and now that He has taken my child; I will never go back!" I said angrily. In my mind, God did not exist. If He did exist, then why is my son dead?

"Yea of little faith." were the words spoken from my Aunt Shirley one Sunday morning. "Get up, clean up, and get dressed for church. I have let you have a pity party for too long. Get up now." she yelled from the kitchen. "God has not done any more to you than He has done to anyone else. You are not the only woman that has loss a child, and you won't be the last." she said loudly. I knew that she was upset, because now she was in my room, standing directly in front of me pointing her finger in my face.

Although I did not want to go to worship, I knew Aunt Shirley was serious. I finally got up, prepared for service, and shortly we were out the door to the church house.

I did not want to be at church. I did not want to look at anyone

,and I did not want anyone looking at me. When I am upset, it will show on my face and through my actions. I did not sing, commune, give, or even pay attention while Bro. Moore was preaching. I had been baptized into the church for 11 years, and even though I knew everything that he preached was truthful, the devil had me right where he wanted me. I could not believe God would put His daughter through this much pain and suffering. My heart was cold as an icebox. For two months, I went through a state of depression. Despite how I felt, God was still good. I wanted to get better, so I started praying fervently for myself. I asked God to help me, and He did. My Aunt Shirley's prayers along with the supplications of the righteous Saints of Delmar Avenue Church of Christ. Those fervent prayers helped me to overcome my battle, and I re-claimed my faith.

I returned to the Lord's house restored. During this test, I learned to have a testimony, you must first have a test; and the teacher is always quiet during the test. It's only God, you and your faith. God can do anything but fail and His hands are too great for mistakes. God tested my every amen and hallelujah, but they were counterfeit. Going forth I would be better equipped, for my storm had transformed me into the person that God needed me to be. My favorite reggae singer, Bob Marley once said, "you never know how strong you are until being strong is your only choice." Being a weak Christian is not an option. Only the strong will survive.

And he saith unto them, why are ye fearful, O ye of little faith? Then he arose, and rebuked the winds and the sea; and there was a great calm.

-Matthew 8:26 (KJV)

Part II

Nine Months Later

Chapter 11

My ex-husband and I apparently thought God was speaking to us, when He said, "be fruitful and multiply." **Nine months later**, we were blessed with another baby boy, which would make child number seven for our union. After losing Baby Jay, I didn't want the same thing to happen again. I was going to try my hardest, so it would not. I made sure I kept every doctor's appointment, and I did exactly what I was told to do. I was considered a high-risk patient because of my previous loss.

There would be days that I felt very little to no movement from the baby, therefore, I was not taking any chances. I went to see my doctor immediately. I refused to lose another child, especially to placental abruption. Although I tried to be optimistic about my pregnancy, I was afraid that I would lose this child too. My doctor was very cautious with my every move. He informed me that placental abruptions often occur suddenly, and there is no hope since the damage has been done.

I knew that to be true since it occurred unexpectedly with Baby Jay.

My First Trimester Screening was performed during the 12th week of my pregnancy. This combination of test would determine if my son would have a birth defects. I'd taken this test during my previous pregnancies; therefore, I wasn't nervous. I was home alone one afternoon, when my cell phone rang. It was my doctor's nurse. "Hello, Tawanda?" she asked politely. "Yes, this is she." I replied. "I am calling because the birth defect tests you took came back today. The numbers used to determine if the child has a birth defect are high, which is not normal. Your baby has spinal bifida." she went on to say.

"WHAT?" I screamed, as I ran out the front door. "Calm down. I have scheduled you an appointment in Jackson for this Friday at 9:00 a.m. to see what is going on with your baby" she stated. "Calm down? You called me with this kind of news, and you expect me to calm down? I yelled louder. I was so hurt. I hung up the phone without a good-bye, and called my Aunt Shirley. I knew she surely would have the words of encouragement that I was so desperately in need of.

I dialed her number, and proceeded to tell her what the nurse had told me. "If something is wrong with the baby, we will help you take care of him. There is nothing you can do about it. Calm down, because God is still good. It could be worst" were her words of comfort. Aunt Shirley defiantly had a way with words.

After talking to her for nearly 10 minutes, I dried the tears that had rolled down my cheeks, walked in house, and pulled out my sonograms.

After having seven children, I had become an expert at reading sonograms. I gathered the 6 pictures of my baby boy, and walked to the kitchen table. I had just had an ultrasound performed a week ago, and the doctor did not mention any abnormalities. I turned the light on, and began to examine the picture closely. I looked at the sonogram of his back for several minutes, and it appeared to be normal to me. I wasn't a professional, but I was comfortable that I was right. As I walked down the hallway to put away the sonograms, "this is a test." ran through my mind. I smiled, prayed, and waited for my Aunt Shirley to come home with my children. Once they arrived home, my aunt and I prayed for a good report from the doctor, since Friday was the next day. I completed my motherly duties, prepared for my trip to Jackson, and went to bed.

The drive to Jackson was hopeful. My ex-husband and I discussed the baby the entire ride. We knew that if we could bury a baby, we could take care of our special needs child if we had to. As soon as we arrived at the hospital, I checked in and waited for the nurse to call us to the examination room. The doctor talked to me about my previous loss, and ensured me that he would not let this baby die. Those words were comfort to my soul.

We arrived at the hospital and remained positive. I signed in and waited for my name to be called. Shortly, I was called to an examination room, and the x-ray technician came in to perform the ultrasound. She instructed me to lie down. She then put the cold Aquasonic 100 Ultrasound Gel on my big round belly. I had learned to read a person's facial expression during the time I loss Baby Jay. You can tell a lot by a person's facial expression. Just looking at her while she was moving the Doppler across my stomach gave me great ease. She was looking strange, but she was shaking her head no. Then suddenly she said, "Nothing is wrong with your baby. He does not have spinal bifida." My ex and I looked at each other with thanksgiving in our hearts. We were deeply relieved. The technician gave me my baby pictures and left.

A few minutes later the doctor came back in. "Everything looks good ma'am. Sometimes these tests can be off. I do not know why your numbers are so high, but your baby is fine." he said. He asked if I wanted to continue to come to Jackson to see him for my prenatal visit, since we had discussed him giving me a C-section at eight months to keep me from having another placental abruption. I believed my doctor back home was good, so I declined. We left the hospital with hopes of having a healthy baby boy in December. Labor Day, three months later, at around 3 'o'clock, I felt no fetal movement. My aunt had finished cooking, so I had eaten and decided to lay down. After eating and drinking something cold, my baby normally moves uncontrollably in my womb. I was nervous as ever. I did not hesitate to call my niece to take me to Indianola to the hospital. By the time, she arrived, I was in excruciating pain, and my contractions were 5 minutes apart. I was in labor. A few months prior, I had threating a miscarriage, but I followed my doctor's orders of complete bed rest, and my chances of having a miscarriage lessened.

We arrived at the hospital, and I was taken directly to labor and delivery. I was hooked up to the baby monitors, so the baby could be monitored. Again, the cold jelly-like substance was applied to my belly, and to no avail; there was no heartbeat. I could not believe nine months later, I had loss another baby. I shook my head in disbelief, while the nurse was yet attempting to find a heartbeat. Without success, she wiped my belly clean and said "I will be right back. I need the doctor." "Okay." I sadly answered. "Here I go again Lord." I thought to myself. I knew my doctor would come in shorty with the "your baby is dead" scenario. To be honest, I did not want to hear it. I wanted this to all be a nightmare, but I could not wake.

He walks in, grabs me by the hand, and breaks the bad news to me. I was emotionless, as tears fell from my face. All I desired to do, was have my baby naturally and in peace. With Baby Jay, I was given the drug Pitocin to speed up my labor, but not this time. I did not want to have my son in a rush. I wanted to bond with him for the last time physically, but I knew he would live in my heart forever. September 5,

2006, I gave birth to a premature, 2 pound 15-ounce unresponsive baby boy, whom I named Jorden De'Shawn. I was positive during my entire pregnancy, but sometimes you must be a realist. That is one of the things I learned from this tribulation. Pray for what you want, but be prepared for the undesired results.

There are somethings that are beyond our control. I thought my son would live if I did everything the doctor ordered, and that was not so. I was not going to lose another child due to placental abruption, I thought; but I did. Though I passed the test of faith, I learned the Bible is true. There was nothing I did that was wrong, but time and chance happens to us all (Ecclesiastes 9:11). My Aunt Shirley came to the hospital, and was amazed. I was sitting in the bed holding my lifeless son. Although I was not happy, I was at peace. I made her heart happy. When it seems there is no way, God always makes a way.

Come to me, all who labor and are heavy laden, and I will give you rest. Take my yoke upon you, and learn from me, for I am gentle and lowly in heart, and you will find rest for your souls. For My yoke is easy, and My burden is light."

-Matthew 11:28-30(NKJV)

The Foundation of the Strom

Chapter 12

I was overwhelmed with a profuse gloom of darkness that dominated my every move. God was with me, but somehow, I felt all alone. My heart was filled with sorrow. I intensely feared the unknown. During the storm, I would learn that fear is one of the most general tricks Satan uses against Christians. To fight this battle effectively, I had to guard my heart and push past the fear of the uncertain by holding to God's unchanging hand. II Timothy 1:7 says; God, has not given us a spirit of fear, but of power and of love and of a sound mind. Reading this scripture daily prepared me for what was to come.

Thursday, March 21, 2013, was day one of our hospital stay at Blair E. Batson Hospital for Children. As the doctors and nurses flooded my brain with information concerning my son, I became overwhelmed. God's grace and mercy were my stepping stones. Having faith in God, and knowing His word gave me great comfort. I meditated on the latter part of Romans 15:4 daily.

For having patience and understanding the scriptures brings unsurpassed comfort, and it gave me hope. I am a child of God, and I was in the biggest storm of my life. Knowing and understanding there is consolation and hope in God's word, I was of good cheer. I had two things I could not loose. FAITH and HOPE.

I was giving a Children's Oncology Group Family Handbook by the oncology social worker. This book helped me to better understand childhood **cancers**, chemotherapy treatment, medical terms, tests, procedures and more. The social worker was very helpful. She gave me the specifics of the hospital and multiple resources. Her help was much needed, for this environment was foreign to me. It was still digesting the fact I was in a hospital and my son was sick.

Although Jay was in the hospital, he did let it get him down. His main concern was getting better and going back to school, so he could graduate. He was a dedicated student. He did not want to get behind on his school assignments. I inquired about the hospital's homebound program. He was given a laptop for school assignments and for recreational use. East Side High was contacted, and his school assignments were faxed weekly. It was difficult getting his assignments faxed to the school, since he wasn't feeling well most days. I decided to put school off until there was a firm diagnosis and treatment had started.

As I was reading the Children's Oncology Handbook, and

mentally preparing myself for the outcome of my son's fate, a radiologist came to perform an x-ray on his heart. The x-ray was done to confirm it was functioning properly before the operation. Blood work, bone and liver scans, and other test were completed throughout the day. These were regular measures, that were taken to ensure he could undergo surgery.

The next day was the day of the surgery. The devil slowly tried to enter my heart, but I prayed him right back to hades. Ja'Marcus and I were praying when the nurses knocked on the door to get him for surgery. I kissed him on his forehead, whispered I love you in his ear, and they proceeded to push him down the hallway. Dr. Carson was the anesthesiologist who put him to sleep and Dr. Zawiya performed the surgery on him at 12:37 PM. Apparently, the devil knew I was not having his drama today, because my heart was fearless during Jay's surgery. I was at peace.

"The procedure went well. There were no issues with him being put to sleep. Three small cuts were made for me to perform the biopsy. He was cut once in his navel, and he has two small incisions on his right side. From looking at the tumor, we believe it to be a germ cell tumor, which is a yolk sac tumor. There are different kind of yolk sac tumors. It will be next week when I know for certain the final diagnosis. A piece of the tumor along with fat from over his bile will be sent to a pathologist to study under a microscope. Freezing, cutting, and staining will also be done on the tumor to get more specific details. Chemotherapy will be needed to treat the **cancer;** therefore, I placed a port-a-cath on the left side of his chest. The port-a-cath is where he will receive chemo, and blood can also be drawn from the port. These tumors respond well to chemotherapy. He will be back to his room once he wakes up." Dr. Zawiya explained. That was a lot of information for me to comprehend, for that reason I am glad I had my tablet and ink pen. "Do you have any questions?" she asked. "Not now." I replied while jotting down what she had already told me. "Thank you." I said, as she left the waiting area.

    She had explained everything so fast, but I understood thus far. I had been reading the book the oncology social worker had given me for about 45 minutes before speaking with the doctor about the germ cell and yolk sac tumor, so I had a little knowledge on what she said. A few hours later, Ja'Marcus was back in his room, and he was in tremendous pain. One of the nurses informed me he had a tumor the size of a grapefruit in his abdomen with many mini tumors. This was one of the reason for the unbearable pain. Not only was his stomach full of tumors, the tumors were producing fluid (ascites) inside his abdomen. During the biopsy, 2 liters of fluid was removed from his stomach. Tiny spots were also found on his lungs. The doctor ensured me once chemotherapy starts, the tumors would stop leaking. The mass was lying low in his abdomen, causing him to produce little to no urine, in addition to having a partial blockage.

    Over the next few days, there were multiple tests, procedures, and scans performed. Ja'Marcus was in constant pain and being in pain was not an option. He had a very high tolerance for pain. Many times, he waited until his pain reached a level 8 or 9 before he would request pain medication. My job was to ensure he was comfortable as possible. Ja'Marcus did not want to take medication day and night. I did not give him a choice because he deserved a quality of life.

Nurse Penny was his favorite nurse. She would talk to him daily to keep his mind occupied. She would come to his room with bags full of goodies every day. She was the best nurse we had encountered at Blair E. Batson Children's Hospital. She made sure that he was well taken care. After I talked to her about his pain, she discussed the matter with Dr. Zawiya. She then ordered he be given Morphine and Percocet around the clock to keep him out of pain. Once the medicine was fully in his system, Ja'Marcus was pain free. I was elated.

I was content with knowing that my son had **cancer**, but my prayers were to let there be a cure. I somehow found myself praying it was a yolk sac tumor. Some of the symptoms he had aligned with this tumor. I just needed confirmation, so I waited patiently. Unfortunately, that was not the case. The day had finally arrived. We waited three long days for the results from the biopsy. There was a light knock at the door. "Come in." I said softly. Dr. Zawiya walked in and greeted my husband and me. I was not aware that tears were flowing down my face. Although I wanted to know the results, I was petrified.

"Mrs. Hudson, the biopsy showed that your son has Hepatocellular Carcinoma. This is a rare and aggressive form of **cancer**. There is currently no known cure." were the words that came out of her mouth. I was speechless. I had no questions because it seemed as if she had predicted my son's future without saying "he is going to die." Thank God Ja'Marcus was asleep. I did not want him to hear such awful news. The remainder of my days in Jackson were miserable. Days had passed, and no one mentioned anything about a treatment plan for my son. Now that I knew there was no cure for his **Cancer**, time was of the essence. I had no time to wait, because his life was on the line.

One morning, I woke up on the wrong side of the bed. As soon as my feet hit the floor, the devil had his way with me. I called my cousin Ann to tell her that we were leaving Jackson. "Where are you going?" she asked. I could not answer her question, as I had no idea where we were going. I ranted about what the doctors, and she quietly listened. As I talked, I packed our belongings. My cousin finally talked some sense into me after a while. I calmed down, gathered my thoughts, and realized I was making an irrational decision, because the only place I had to go was home. Home was not an option because my son needed immediate medical attention. "Do you know what stage the **Cancer** is in?" she asked. "No, I don't want to know." I said in low tone. "You need to know. Get off the phone and go ask the doctor" she said. When I finished talking to my cousin, all our bags were packed, and I was ready to go. I just didn't know where I was going.

Apart of me wanted to know what stage my child's **cancer** was in, but another part of me did not. I wrestled with the thoughts of questioning the doctor for nearly an hour. I eventually build up the courage to ask. I slowly opened Ja'Marcus' room door and walked to the desk where one of the doctors who worked with Dr. Zawiya was sitting. As I walked down the hall, my legs were shaking as if I had seen a ghost. "Excuse me sir. I have a question. What stage is my son's **cancer**?" I asked with a trembling voice. He was on the phone, and he asked the person on the phone to "politely" hold on. "Oh, your son's **cancer** is in stage 4." he replied with no sorrow.

My eyes bucked, and I hit the floor as if I had been knocked out by Mike Tyson. I woke up in the lobby with my husband fanning me. I was crying uncontrollably. Once I settled down a nurse assisted my husband with walking me back to Jay's room since I was weak. My blood pressure was elevated, and I could hardly think straight. The way I was feeling, I could have been the patient. Minutes later Nurse Penny came to the room, to empty Jay's Foley catheter bag, and I inquired about his treatment. "All oncologists, radiologists, surgeons, radiation oncologists, pathologists, nurses and social workers will have a meeting on Wednesday. They will come up with a treatment plan for Ja'Marcus then." she stated as she left the room.

The rude doctor I had talked to earlier walked into the room shortly after Nurse Penny left. Without a knock at the door, he let himself in. I was already mad, and his actions made me madder. He had no bed-side manners. I pondered where our primary doctor was, so I asked, "Where is Dr. Zawiya? "She will no longer be working with your son. I am his new oncologist Dr. Jumar." he said with a thick accent. I shook my head in disbelief. "Lord, be a fence around me." I mumbled. I was under enough stress. I was not going to allow an impolite doctor to add to it. I checked for his grade on Healthgrades.com, and he did not have one. After observing his foul behavior, I understood why. In my book, no grade meant he had a zero.

He explained the children's oncologists wanted to be sure my son diagnosis of Hepatocellular Carcinoma was correct. They needed my permission to give the biopsy results to the adult oncologists to read for a second opinion. I had a sense of relief with knowing Jay may not have this aggressive form of **cancer**. I quickly agreed, and he rushed the results to adult oncologists. The same afternoon, an oncologist came to speak with me concerning their finding. The **cancer** Dr. Jumar and Zawiya believed it to be, the adult oncologists said the mass appeared to be a different form **cancer**. That was my que. It was defiantly time for us to go.

While the doctors seemed to be at a standstill, I was busy looking for my son a hospital that could give him more than a pill to buy him a few more months of life. Yes, this was the approach the medical team planned for my son. Nexavar or generically known as Sorafenib, is a chemotherapy drug used to treat kidney, liver, and thyroid **Cancer**. This was the hope they offered us. I thought about St. Jude Children's Research Hospital because Jermaine had mentioned it a few days earlier. I used the computer the oncologist social worker had given Ja'Marcus to fill out the refer a patient application for St. Jude. When she came back to the room later in the day, I gave her the computer to complete the form by adding Dr. Jumar's doctor credentials. She did not hesitate to complete the application, emailing the scans, and mailing the biopsy results, to St. Jude Children's Research Hospital. Scottish Rite and Emory Children's Center were hospitals I had considered taking Ja'Marcus to in Atlanta. I had given the social worker the phone number and contact person for each facility. Like with St. Jude, she sent everything that was needed to have my son transferred without delay. The way things were at this point, I was going to the hospital who contacted me first. ***The foundation of the storm*** had begun.

"There are some things you can only learn in a storm."

Alternative Holistic Treatment
Chapter 13

I wanted my son to live more than anything on earth. Since the doctors could not help him to live, I had too. I was desperate for a cure and desperate times cause for desperate measures. I decided to try an **alternative holistic treatment** plan. I spoke with a gentleman whose love one had undergone this form of treatment. Since it helped him to live a few extra years, I felt that it was worth a try. Holistic treatment is a form of remedies that tries to treat the patient on diverse levels. This technique of healing looks at the well-being, emotionally, physically, spiritually, and mentally before a treatment plan is given.

There was no harm in trying a natural approach. I was given the name and phone number of a holistic doctor from the Jackson area. He made natural medications especially for **cancer** patients. I contacted Mr. London with no hesitation. He gave me told me information an oncologist would never say. "**Cancer** is a state of health, and not a state of illness" he said. He believed Ja'Marcus' immune system had failed, and it simply needed to be repaired. He asked me several questions about my son's spiritual life, medical condition, stress level, diet, and sleep pattern, in order that he could gather the appropriate medicines that would keep the **cancer** from spreading more and cause his immune system to work properly. He gave me his address, and my husband went to meet him. I prayed while he was gone, because I really needed God to work through these medications.

While Jermaine was gone, I called my cousin to let her know what I was preparing to do. She thought it was a good idea to try it, but I needed to search the medications before giving them to him. Jermaine walked through the door while I was on the phone. He handed me a bag full of medicine. I took the bag, opened it and began sorting out the bottles. As I sorted them out, I told my cousin the name of each one. She wrote down the name the pills with the intention of researching it later.

I did not wait for her to find facts regarding the treatment, for I was in a hurry to start administering the meds to him. During this time, Google became my best friend. I studied each medication for hours. My main consideration was the side effects. Although I wanted my son to live, I did not want to harm him in the process. Mr. London had given me seven bottles of pills, a bottle of oil and a liquid medication to administer to my son around the clock. However, there were more negative side effects than positive for most of them. There were two pills I assumed Ja'Marcus would benefit from, so I gave them to him for nearly a two week. Ja'Marcus initially was fine with this form of treatment, but after a few days, he decided he did not want to take the pills anymore. I found this to be bizarre, because by some means during the same time, I wasn't as enthused at this point as I was when I first spoke with Mr. London concerning the medication. A cluster of fear had activated inside of me. I did not want to make bad matters worse, especially since he'd started to vomit profusely from taking the pills. I followed my first mind and stopped the holistic treatment.

Inwardly I felt as if God was taking too long. I wanted my child to be healed. I had to take matters into my own hands and heal him. Wait! What was I thinking? I instantaneously slowed down and realize I had no power over this. I was not God. Who was I to rush Him? Whenever He came, He would surely be on time. The Bible has a way of comforting one's soul. I was reminded of Psalm 30:2, Lord my God, I called you for help, and you healed me. God had already calmed the sea, I just had to go through the storm. Even if it be through death, the storm is over. The body can only achieve what the heart believes, and Yahweh was inscribed in my soul. Jesus heals.

"Children are the anchors of a Mother's heart."

In the Mist of the Storm
Chapter 14

I would walk through the chilling waters *in the mist of the storm*, feeling as if I was going to drown. I felt the massive rush of the wind beating upon me, but I had no doubts, for Jehovah God was with me. I prayed to him zealously, and it was then I recognized it was safe for me to let go and let God.

Our time in Jackson, at Blair E. Batson Hospital for Children had expired. While my son and I built a relationship with the oncology staff, there was no hope for him there. As we walked further into the storm, I continued to hold God's.

St. Jude Children's Research Hospital sent an ambulance for my son and I on April 2, 2013. Before leaving Blair E. Batson Hospital for Children, I kneeled to Jesus before telling Ja'Marcus snippets of his condition. I wanted to protect him as best as I could. For that reason, I did not tell him the severity of the **Cancer**. Him knowing that he had **Cancer** was enough, in my opinion. When I spoke with the oncologists concerning his condition, I stood in the hallway. I could not bring myself to tell him there was no cure for his disease. I did not want to see the fear on his face and I did not want him to worry. I cringed with the idea of him fearing he'd die.

The drive to Memphis was long, tedious, and bumpy. Ja'Marcus and I chatted to liven up the ride. The EMTs heard Jay and I talking about sports, and they joined the conversation. Ja'Marcus was a true sports fan, so their conversation kept him woke the entire ride. They laughed and told jokes about each other favorite team. This made my heart glad, given that it helped both of us to take our minds off reality for a while. I sat there silently and listened to them talk, since I have no knowledge of sports.

The EMTs stopped to get gas, and they thought it would be wise for Ja'Marcus to use the restroom since we had another hour to travel. They went above and beyond the call of duty to ensure that he was happy and stress-free. I went inside the store to get snacks at Jay's request. This was an inspiring moment, since he hadn't had an appetite since we'd been in Jackson. I walked out the store, and waited for Jay and the EMTs to come out. Moments later, they were heading back to the ambulance laughing and talking. They assisted Jay back on the ambulance, gassed up, and we were off to St. Jude.

We arrived at the emergency entrance at St. Jude Children's Research Hospital at 12:30 PM. The two EMTs opened the back doors of the ambulance, and helped Ja'Marcus to get out. He had enough strength to walk, so they allowed him to do so, with their assistance. It felt good to see him walking, because he had been extremely weak. There were several nurses waiting on our arrival. I gladly walked alongside my son, the nurses and EMTs as we headed to the admission department of the hospital. I was in a peaceful state of mind the entire trip to Memphis. The devil seemed to know we'd arrived at the hospital, since my soul unexpectedly became vexed. My mind rendered negative thoughts by the second. I knew it was time for me to go to God in prayer. If anyone can fix a broken situation, Jesus can.

Walking down the halls of St. Jude Children's Research Hospital, I felt a sincere and inviting essence. This was a feeling I did not feel during our stay in Jackson. We were instantly caressed with love from the staff instantaneously. Ja'Marcus' face appeared to be peaceful, and he seemed to have a relaxed since of comfort. Once we made it to admissions one of the EMTs prayed for us, wished us well, and departed.

I was given a countless number of papers to read and sign during admission, in addition to answering several questions. We were given a tour of the hospital, and information on what to expect during every out and inpatient visit. "I like St. Jude!" Ja'Marcus said excitedly. Coming here truly seemed to do him well because while we were touring the hospital, he asked the tour guide, "where is the cafeteria?" His appetite was coming back, and personally that was a good sign since he was scarcely eating at Batson.

We walked to Kay's Café, where he purchased a grilled chicken sandwich, french fries and a Gatorade with the meal card that he was given by the admission clerk. Shortly after the tour, Jay's room was cleaned, and he was ready for what was next.

The news we'd received in Jackson was disheartening. It crushed me to my lowest point, but being skeptical of what God can do and giving up was not an option. For God had his back spiritually. I had his back physically. I was going to be strong for my son because he needed me. Our journey on earth is temporary, but to die and live with the Lord is eternal life. I prayed my son would live, yet if he died, he will die a child of the Master.

Ja'Marcus, if I had to choose between loving you and breathing...I would use my last breath to tell you...
I LOVE YOU!

Walking Through the Storm by Faith
Chapter 15

I was constantly faced with the unknown, but I continued **walking through the storm by faith**. Faith is letting God have absolute control even when you don't know the outcome. It wasn't easy and I won't pretend it was. Even though I had great uncertainties, worrying about what was to come would not benefit me or help the situation. Knowing that God was present made my burdens lighter

We met the medical team we'd be working with at St. Jude at D Clinic. D Clinic is for patients who have solid tumors. I was in complete awe at how much kindness they showed to us. "This is an amazing children's institute" I thought. Here, the children are top priority. They ensure the parent has one primary concern, their child. I had no bigger joy than recognizing my son was in first-class care.

In the beginning, I did not want my son to know the severity of his condition, because I did not want him to worry. Dr. Elise did not agree with me. "This is his body. He deserves to know what is going on in his body. It is not fair to him" she said.

I could not question her since she was right. I just wanted to protect him from being hurt. Once Ja'Marcus learned the full extinct and severity of his condition, he was blank. He had no words neither did he did complain. He never worried. He truly allowed God to fight his battle because he instantly went to God in prayer. "I am going to be fine" were his words always.

Dr. Sidney and Dr. Freeman were the first oncologists from D Clinic that we met. Along with the fellow, Dr. Elise who worked faithfully alongside Dr. Freeman. We worked with Dr. Sidney for a short period since she basically confirmed my son's diagnosis. They'd already received Ja'Marcus' information from the children's oncologists in Jackson, and their findings were correct. The **cancer** was stage IV Hepatocellular Carcinoma. Hepatocellular carcinoma is a form of liver **cancer** that typically affects people whose livers have been under extra stress for an extended period because of continued use of drugs, metabolic diseases, or infections. The **cancer** started in his liver and it had metastasized to his lungs. Being this **cancer** was rare, there was no cure, but it could be treated. I was told by one doctor, he'd never seen this kind of **cancer** during his career as an oncologist. Hearing this frightening me even more, but where there is a will, there is a way.

Ja'Marcus was blessed to meet a young man name Maximillian Burdette at the 2013 annual prom held at St. Jude, and they became close friends.

They were the only two patients who had the same **cancer** at St. Jude, but their bond was deeper than **cancer**. They now had someone to talk with, a person who understood their everyday feelings. Having someone to communicate with, eased the stress of their lives. I was blessed to meet Max's mother Christiana. We became good friends, with an everlasting bond. We understood one another's pain just as our sons did. We talked, we laughed, and we cried together. Despite what the doctors had said, we continued to look for the good in a bad situation. Desmond Tutu once said, "hope is being able to see that there is light despite all of the darkness." Our path was dark as a cloudy night with no view of the stars or moon, but we had our spiritual light, Jesus.

    After the doctors did their research, I was given a treatment plan before we left to go home. There were three chemotherapy drugs that were generally used to treat the **cancer**, along with several solid tumor clinical trials. All treatments may or may not help to shrink or stabilize the tumor. The primary drug Ja'Marcus was prescribed was the pill the oncologist in Jackson told me about, Nexavar or Sorafenib. This **cancer** drug is used to hinder the growth and spread of **cancer** cells in the patient's body. Cisplatin and Doxorubicin are other drugs that would be given intravenously. Cisplatin would be infused with Mannitol and run over six hours. He would also get a bag of Mannitol before the Cisplatin treatment. Mannitol is used to make one urinate and keep the kidneys from shutting down.

Doxorubicin was the red bag of chemo, and it was sensitive to light. After waiting an hour after the Cisplatin was given, the Doxorubicin would then be administered. Adavan, Dexathason, Ondansetron, Benadryl, and Zofran, are a few of the nausea medications that he would be given after the Cisplatin because chemo normally makes one nauseous. Ja'Marcus was not eligible for a liver transplant since the **Cancer** had spread. His only chance of survival was surgery. The chemo will not dissolve the tumors completely, but with hope they will shrink, then the oncologists could consider surgery.

Nonetheless, we were please, since previously we had very little expectations of treatment. I'd learned to let God lead me in making decisions. Hence, we prayed and opt for the first chemotherapy we were offered which is known as combination therapy. We'd digest the diagnosis, now we had to ingest getting treatment. Ja'Marcus and I both had blended feelings of happiness and sadness while he was preparing for his first round of chemo. It had been several days since the biopsy and the placement of the port-a-cath, and the thoughts of finally getting treatment was a huge relief for us both.

My son was taking several pills a day. The thought of me learning how to administer his medication caused me to panic. Before we left to go home, Ja'Marcus' favorite male nurse took me to Pharmacy to pick up his medication. He explained to me what I should do when I needed to pick up medication.

"How am I supposed to learn all of this" I asked him. "Trust me, you will get the hang of it. After doing it a few times, you will be a supermom" he said. He sure did tell the truth. I was very organized. I put all his medication in a bag. I labeled the top of each bottle with the name and time he should be given the medicine. This way, I ensured that he took his medication on time every day. Although it was not required, I took his temperature daily. I was being on the safe side. If he had a temperature of 100.4, we were encouraged to go to St. Jude immediately. Ja'Marcus meant everything to me. I could not fail him. He needed me and I needed him. I was going to be right by his side until the end.

The journey wasn't filled with butterflies and tulips every day. There were days I was knocked down with bad news, but God allowed me to get up and smile although I was dying inside from heartache and pain.

Ja'Marcus could go home for two weeks before chemotherapy began since he was stable, and his pain was controlled. This gave him and his siblings time to bond since they'd been separated for nearly two months. They were excited to see one another as it was written all over their faces. Jay loved his siblings, but he and his baby sister Skylar shared a unique relationship. It was amazing watching them interact.

It was a sad moment to see the kids say their goodbyes, but we had to part ways for a while. Ja'Marcus was anxious to get his treatments started, so he could "be a normal kid" again. Hearing him say those words, put a sad essence in my spirit. **Cancer** was not in my plans for my child's future. I hated he was going through this pain and agony. I talked to God, and prayerfully we would soon be back home, and things would be normal. I walked to the admission clerk's desk at St. Jude and gave her Jay's medical record number, 39392. After which, we were given his inpatient wrist band, and headed to triage. Once we were done in triage, we were escorted to Ja'Marcus' room where we were ready for chemo.

Now faith is the substance of things hoped for, the evidence of things not seen.

-Hebrews 11:1(KJV)

Expect the Unexpected
Chapter 16

Chemo was completed, and I was right by Ja'Marcus' bedside, like always. I had buzzed the nurse for his dose of Zofran since he was vomiting profusely. He was asleep yet in a lethargic state. The doctors did not warn me about him being lethargic, therefore, I was somewhat alarmed. I had never seen him this way. He was trying to speak, but his speech was slurred, and he had abnormal eye movement. The nurse and I spoke with the oncologists and they too found it to be out of the ordinary. They'd never witnessed this type of behavior after any chemo treatment. They waited to see how he'd be the next day, but tomorrow brought no change.

It hurt me to the core to see my son in the condition he was in. There was nothing I could do to help him physically, but spiritually I called out to God on his behalf. God placed me in a situation, where I had to fully rely on him. There is this saying, "when life knocks you to your knees, you're in a good position to pray; and that is just what I did; prayed.

The next morning, Ja'Marcus had stopped vomiting, but the lethargic state had worsened. The doctors were baffled. They ordered he be taken off all medications that cause drowsiness right away. Dr. Freeman and Dr. Elise came to check on him the next morning hoping he would be better. Since his condition had not improved, a CT scan of his brain was ordered. The nurses soon came to take him to the Department of Diagnostic Imaging for scans.

Ja'Marcus was asleep until it was time for the scans. Once the radiologist proceeded to help the nurses to get him out of the hospital bed, Ja'Marcus became infuriated. He was disoriented and agitated. He was striking everyone who tried to touch him. Nurses and doctors from other floors were paged to help control him. It took six people to hold him down. He was screaming, attempting to tell us something, but no one could understand a word he said. Now since he was trying to pull the lines of his port out, he had to be restrained. There was nothing I could do for my son beside pray. I was completely helpless.

Once they could control him, he was taken back to the room. His doctors were quickly updated on what had occurred. Dr. Elise ordered a Complete Blood Count. Since doing the CT scan was not successful, she was sure this would give her a clue of what may be going on. Ja'Marcus had now calmed down and was asleep.

The day seemed long as I waited for the results. Ja'Marcus was restless since he struggled to take the restraints off several times. Words cannot describe how I felt, as I tighten the loosen restraints. My child knew every nurse and doctor that cared for him, now he recognized no one, not even me. A praying mother is more valuable than every diamond in the world. Therefore, I prayed for my son until I dozed off into a light sleep. Prayer has a way of soothing a weary soul.

The nurse came in and woke me up with the CBC results. Everything appeared to good, except his ammonia level was over 600. Ammonia is natural waste produced in the body. It comes from absorbing protein by bacteria in one's intestines. If the ammonia is not managed by the liver and removed from the body appropriately, too much ammonia will build up in the blood and transfer from the blood to the brain, where it now can lead to a coma, brain damage, and death.

Ja'Marcus had been in a coma for about 2 days when the doctors decided to nasal intubate him. Since Ja'Marcus was combative with the medical team, it took several people to hold him down to complete the procedure. Ja'Marcus begin to vomit, so the procedure didn't go as anticipated. By some means the tubes came through his mouth and he begin to choke. Once he'd stopped vomiting, they were able to put the tubes in. Chinney was upset and fearful since he had to see his brother go through such distress. I cried hysterically as I tried to console Chinney.

The doctors and nurses were moving like bolts of lightning in and out of Ja'Marcus' room. My body was numb since they had put me out, so I watched from the parent's room which was beside Ja'Marcus' room.

I was getting a spiritual beating, and the carnal side of me was ready to tap out. I was weak as water, but I knew somebody who was strong, Aunt Shirley. I grabbed my cell phone and called her, because I needed a quick dose of reality. If anyone would give it to me straight, it would be her. I explained to her what was going on and these were her words, "Your son may die, but your son is no better than anyone else's son. How old is he? He is 17. The Lord allowed you to know him longer than Jay and Jorden. You knew them only in your womb. The good thing about this all is he is a Christian and God is still good." Our conversation ended abruptly since Aunt Shirley had absolutely no filter when it came to painting the real picture of life. Her words were appalling, but I meditated on what she'd said until they had finished intubating my son. The more I thought about her words, the more I realized she was right. My Aunt Margaret told me to always ***expect the unexpected***, but I certainly was not expecting this. The doctors believed he would be the coma indefinitely because he showed no signs of improvement, but God saw differently. I thought to myself, "could life get any worse?"

> I have seen something else under the sun: The race is not to the swift or the battle to the strong, nor does food come to the wise or wealth to the brilliant or favor to the learned; but time and chance happeneth to them all.
>
> -Ecclesiastes 9:11 (NIV)

A Storm Inside a Storm

Chapter 17

Crying became a part of me. When I thought, I couldn't shed another tear, here comes more bad news, which brought more sobbing. My heart was as heavy as a ton of bricks. How much more could I take? I felt as if I was nearing my breaking point, but breaking was not an option. I had to be there for my son. I promised him at birth I would always be by his side, and only death would break my promise. Going through the storm was tough. I had to put on the whole armor of God, because my storm's strength had the force of tornadic winds. I was being tossed to and fro, but I continued to weather the storm for I knew a sunshine was bound to shine again.

Ja'Marcus was diagnosed with a genetic disorder, known as Urea Cycle Disorder or UCD, which is a metabolic abnormality. Dr. Elise explained genetic factors give the body commands on how it must breakdown protein. Oftentimes, UCD is detected at birth, but not in our case. Ja'Marcus was a healthy child. One symptom he had that was related to UCD was vomiting.

As soon as I changed his formula, the vomiting ended. Urea Cycle Disorder is caused by a modification that brings about an absence in one of the six enzymes in the urea cycle. The enzyme Ja'Marcus lack was the ornithine transcarbamylase enzyme or OTC. These enzymes are accountable for eliminating ammonia from the blood stream. Since my son lacked the OTC enzymes, over the years his liver worked hard to function, it became stressed, and resulting in **cancer**. Unfortunately, there is no cure for UCD.

Ja'Marcus was given the drug Laxulose to help lower the level of ammonia in his blood, but this was a slow process. The oncologist from St. Jude soon collaborated with the experts on UCD at LeBonheur Children's Hospital, in Memphis to find a treatment plan for him. After a series of test, he was prescribed Glycerol Phenylbutyrate or Ravicti. Ja'Marcus was the only child at St. Jude taking this medication since his illness is rare. He responded well to the Ravicti. After several days, his ammonia levels began to decrease. Ja'Marcus' favorite male nurse was in his room checking his vital signs, when he woke up, and suddenly said, "will you take these restraints off." He was shocked, and I was happy the old Ja'Marcus had returned. From this point, his ammonia levels were monitored closely, but it was no guarantee his levels would not rise again.

Weeks later, before 6 o'clock in the morning, I was watching the news. I woke up and checked on Ja'Marcus throughout the night to ensure he was comfortable since he'd had chemo a few hours earlier.

Ja'Marcus was attempting to get up but he was confused. I knew right away what the problem was. I immediately buzzed for his nurse. His levels were checked, and it was over 400. Like the first episode, he had to be restrained. This time, he was in a coma longer than before. Dr. Freeman and Dr. Elise along with Ja'Marcus' neurologist Dr. Zola became extremely concerned after he was in a coma for 4 days. They then placed orders for a series of blood test and a CT scan of his brain. An electroencephalogram (EEG) was ordered to determine if he was having seizures.

The EEG showed no seizure activity. Since he was showing no signs of improvement he was intubated and put in ICU. Again, we were at a point of no hope. I was advised by his medical team to contact the family, because he may not wake up. I without delay contacted our immediate family and members of the church. Dr. Elise had a gentle heart. She believed his father should be aware of what was going on as well. Our feelings were not mutual. I only agreed to contact him because of the Jesus that dwells in me, not because he deserved the father of the year award. If he was concerned about his son, hell in hot water would not have kept him away. His father had been to the hospital one time since his son had been admitted and that was for less than an hour.

I couldn't contact Ja'Marcus' father, so I called his grandmother (his father's mother). I told her who I was and what the physicians had told me about her grandson's declining health.

She ensured me she would let his father know I'd called and she did. Days later, his father arrived at St. Jude where he stayed for three days. Being the mother of an ill child was no walk in the park, but being the father of an ill child gave me the impression it was like eating a slice of cake. Leaving the hospital was never an option for me, while his dad came and went as he pleased. He would say, "I hate to see him like that." Did he think I signed up to watch my son suffer? I did not want to see him in that condition, but I had no other choice. That was my child lying in the hospital bed, and leaving his side was never a choice.

Another EEG along with other test was performed on him by Dr. Zola, and he seemed to be doing well. Four days after his father left, he woke up. It would have made his heart glad to wake up and see his dad. Nonetheless, like always; I was right as he looked for me. My eyes were full of tears as he stared at me, smile, and gave me a thumb up. Me being strong is an understatement because it wasn't me. It was all God. He was taking me through a storm, but despite how low I sometimes felt, He was still there. Just as He calmed the sea in Matthew 8:23-27, one day, someday, the storm would cease.

Did my son's father and I cause his unfortunate illness? I beat myself up because someone had to take the blame. I carried him for nine months. Place the blame on me. I am the reason my child is sick and I am the reason my child will die of **cancer**. I will never forgive myself for killing my own child. What kind of mother am I?

The devil placed these doubtful thoughts in my heart. It is Satan's goal for a child of God to turn their back on Him especially in the time of trouble, but that was not going to happen. God was the reason I had made it this far. I cried, as I flooded heaven with prayers on behalf of my son. I was in *a storm inside a storm*, but I had the best lifeguard possible, JESUS.

Consider it pure joy, my brothers and sisters, whenever you face trials of many kinds, because you know that the testing of your faith produces perseverance.

– James 1:2-3 (NIV)

What is Family?
Chapter 18

What is family? According to Webster, a family is a basic social unit consisting of parents and their children whether dwelling together or not. I oftentimes say family is a group of people God has given us. We had no personal say in choosing these group of people. Families should share a special bond, but that is not always the case. Relatives should have a Ford tough relationship. There should be an ultimate pact to love, cherish, and protect one another. These individuals are to morally be there for each other through thick and thin. There's a saying, "blood is thicker than water." Although in the physical sense this statement is true, but there are friends that will be there when family is not. According to the scriptures, there is a friend that will stick closer than a brother (Proverbs 18:24). No family is perfect. There will be occasional disputes, but this should never cause division amongst them.

Storms are designed to be a blessing in our lives, for they pave the way for where the Lord wants us to be. In the storm,

God is teaching us what He know we need to become a better person. It is up to us to determine what that something is and use it in our daily walk with Him. It is imperative for you to know who should be allowed in your life and who should not. People enter our lives for a reason and sometimes a season. You have seasonal people and there are permanent people. Seasonal people are meant to journey in your life for a short while, for where God is leading you, they cannot journey. While, permanent people will stand a lifetime. These people are strong, resembling the root of a tree. These are the people you want to hold on to since they are rare. They can come in the form of family or friends. During my son's illness, I found out the permanent and seasonal individuals. Letting go of certain people wasn't easy, but it was best for me as a Christian, and unfortunately, most of those people I called "family."

St. Jude is in the heart of Memphis, Tennessee, which happens to be my birthplace. My mother, step-father, and siblings live there in addition to other "supposedly" relatives. I knew without a doubt my son and I would have a great family support system, and for the most part we did. My immediate family was there from the beginning, but there was a turning point and I began looking at family slightly different. I learned the true meaning of family during my son's first coma.

We have family members who live in Memphis and they never came to visit us.

They never called or thought enough of us to send a quick "how's things going" text message. This was a trying time, and without a doubt I knew these people would have been there, but boy was I wrong. People in the community in which I live, supported us more than relatives that lived blocks away. A countless number of Ja'Marcus' childhood friends were nowhere to be found during his illness. There were several young men and a "so-called cousin", whom he was very acquainted with, they too never visited. He mentioned this to me on several occasions. "Momma, the children at East Side care more for me than the kids I went to school with in Ruleville." I cried for I was heartbroken, but with a bold voice I stated, "don't worry about the ones that aren't here, be grateful for the people that are."

Without a father, a child cannot be created, therefore fathers have an important role within the family. A father should not merely be a man that creates a child, but his job is to nurture, protect and love his child regardless. I knew the consequences of having a child out of wedlock and I firmly understood the choice I'd made. Ja'Marcus was created out of iniquity and lust. Although my child was not a sin, my actions were. From birth, I vowed to my son I would be by his side come rain or shine. I was going to protect him from anyone and anything that would possibly cause him harm and heartache, including his father.

When Ja'Marcus' father decided he did not want to be a part of his life, I was 18 years old.

I was a young adult, but I took his decision with a grain of salt. I could have stooped to his level of immaturity, but I was a mother. His juvenile actions were not going to affect how I reared my child. One thing I knew for certain, my little boy was going to have a good life.

My son walked passed his father on multiple occasions and no words were exchanged. He knew our son existed, but my son did not know he existed. I shield him from his father, not because I wanted to but because at the time it was the best thing for him. I refused to allow him to walk in and out of my child's life at his request.

Two years later, I met and married Ja'Marcus' younger siblings father. Ja'Marcus knew him as being his father until the age of 13. However, as Ja'Marcus continued to grow older, he matured into a mirror image of his dad. Now that it was becoming more evident that he was my son's father, without a DNA test; he began to pay child support. Really? What a slap in the face! I'd taken care of my son with the help of my grandmother and aunts for years. I did not need his bi-weekly $60. My son was in middle school, what was $120 a month going to do for him? Children need their father's presence, not just their monthly donation. However, he believed that paying child support was enough. No visits and limited phone calls was the treatment he gave me son. Not once did I question his actions. I knew and fully understood at a young age, a father is a man that will go above and beyond for his children. Ja'Marcus was in the 7th grade when his father decided to "man up."

Although his "manning up" limited him to be a part time father, Ja'Marcus wanted to get to know him, therefore, I allowed him to create a bond with his dad. My father passed away before I was born, and I wanted to know him. Therefore, I knew it was vital my son developed a relationship with his father.

After Ja'Marcus was diagnosed with **cancer**, it was months before I informed his father. Why? This man had done nothing for his son during the 16 years he was healthy. What could he possibly do for him now, since he'd been diagnosed with a terminal illness? Exactly...**ABSOLUTLEY NOTHING**! After he learned that his child was sick, he came to visit him four times. The first visit lasted nearly an hour, but this visit meant so much to Ja'Marcus for he and his father had never sat down and had a real father son conversation. Unfortunately, the conversation was basically concerning his battle with **cancer**. During the last visit, he did not want to come inside the house. If his son needed him at any point, it was during this time since he was in the first phase of transitioning. I couldn't be mad with him, because I expected this behavior. I'd dealt with his immatureness my son's entire life. It was nothing new.

I can't help but to ponder the thoughts, "how could a father be so cold-hearted towards his own seed?" "How could he say he loved him, yet never displayed his love for him?" "How could he allow his child to be birthed into the world without him and to die without him?"

His son was slowing expiring, but he assumed it was appropriate to send the neighborhood's drug dealer by to check on "his" child. I WAS BEYOND FERIOUS!!!!!! Since he used my son as an alibi to miss work, the least he could have done was to call and check on him. What kind of man does this, especially to his dying child? I'll tell you what kind of man does that. A man that should not have been a father from the start. A family cannot be stronger than a parent and child. Although my son's father did not live with him, he is still his family. Even in death, but he saw differently.

My husband is thee absolute BEST! He stepped up to rear seven children that are not biologically his. He wasn't merely by my side when Ja'Marcus became ill, but he was right there until the very end. He and Ja'Marcus shared a special father-son bond. They shared a bond that he did not share with his biological father, therefore, I will never label him as being my children's stepfather, but he is their father.

Life's definition of family is that person that will go an extra mile for you, a person that is there when you need them most. A person that is willing to make sacrifices for you. During this time, my son learned who his real family and friends were. People that he knew should have been there, but they were not. I knew inwardly this hurt him, but I always reminded him that if he had no other earthly being, he had me. I was there from birth and I will be there until death. I am my son's definition of family.

How could family act in such a manner? These are not just random people. These are close relatives and friends. Individuals that we've known for a lifetime. People whom we thought we had a strong bond with. We called them family, but their actions displayed that of a foe. After entering my prayer closet multiple times; I forgave them, and I now count it all joy. I learned a lifelong lesson in the storm. It doesn't matter how long you've known a person or your relationship status with a person; people change. Trust God, because putting too much trust in man is a treacherous thing. People have the capability to deceive, but God will never forsake you (Hebrews 13:5). Family doesn't have to be blood-related, but they must be real.

The bond I shared with my son was nothing short of amazing. Everything I did for him, was out of love and because I carried him for nine months. I was his biggest supporter. If I had to do it all over again, I would.

"You don't choose your family. They are God's gift to you, as you are to them."

Desmond Tutu

The Best News Ever

Chapter 19

I later learned Cisplatin contains a high amount of ammonia, therefore Jamarcus' ammonia level would increase after chemo. This was an excessive amount of ammonia in his body to remove, since he had a metabolic disorder. He would no longer use the combination chemo Doxorubicin and Cisplatin. He was now a candidate for a trial treatment of chemo. Doxorubicin and Cisplatin kept the **cancer** stable. My hopes were for the trial chemo to shrink the mass. I continued to go to God in prayer for He was my primary source of help. My son's **Cancer** had not been cured, but I continued to look beyond the mountains. I had hope.

A few weeks after each round of chemo, a CT scan was performed. The new scans are compared to the previous scans, and this determines if the **cancer** was stable or if it had grown. Being scheduled to have scans was always a dreadful time for me. I hated to see the expression of my child's face, particularly if it was bad news. I had learned to read his doctor's actions.

If they walked in with small talk, I knew the results were bad. If they came in and immediately gave me the results, it was good news, the mass had either shrunk or it was stable.

The first chemotherapy did not reduce the size of the **cancer**, instead the **cancer** grew and my son experienced alopecia for the first time. Consequently, the doctors decided to try another trial chemo with our approval. After having five rounds of the clinical trial chemo and having no change; I was overwhelmed. I sat in the lobby of D Clinic and cried until I couldn't shed another tear. "Don't cry Momma. I am going to try another chemo. I will be fine" were the words my courageous son stated. I was supposed to console him, yet once again, he was comforting me. Ja'Marcus was on the new chemo for almost two months, and it was working. It had reduced the size of the tumors tremendously. Our hearts were ecstatic.

If Ja'Marcus felt fine, I continued to work. I was on lunch break one evening, when Dr. Freeman called me with *the best news ever*. This was the best news I'd heard since his diagnosis. "Ja'Marcus' tumors have shrunk enough to have surgery. This is his only chance of survival; so, I have scheduled him an appointment to meet with surgeon Dr. Denali right away. He will answer all your questions. Good luck" he said. After I wrote down the surgeon's name, phone number, and address, I gladly said "thank you and goodbye." I called Ja'Marcus and told him the wonderful news. We both wept with tears of happiness after which Ja'Marcus prayed and we ended our conversation. God was boldly walking in the storm with me and I could feel His presence.

"Life isn't about waiting for the storm to pass. It's learning to pray in the rain."

Time for Surgery
Chapter 20

I found it ironical that the ribbon color for liver **cancer** is emerald green and it represents hope. This was amazing news for us, since Ja'Marcus and I wore green constantly before learning this. There were three things we held close to my heart, God, faith, and hope.

After the initial appointment with Surgeon Denali at his Germanton office, we were filled with excitement. Granting everything he said was not positive, a true solider always remains optimistic. We had come too far for doubts. When a storm is nearing, other birds seek shelter, but the eagle flies beyond the storm. It does not escape the storm, it simply uses the storm to elevate. I had to be like an eagle. There was no way of escaping, so I allowed my tribulation to push me higher than my storm, this only meant I was closer to God.

Dr. Denali had a heartfelt spirit. He was a physician like no other. He displayed great empathy towards my son.

Simply listening to him, it was obvious he cared wholeheartedly. It is rare to find a doctor that shares your pain as a parent, and for him I was appreciative. He gave us hope like no other medical professional had. He was straight forward with me concerning my son's prognosis. Although he had looked at the scans of Ja'Marcus' abdomen, he and his partner would not know the extinct of the **cancer** until he actually cut him open. He made no promises or guarantees, but he said, "I am going to try my best to get all the **cancer** out of his belly. I have a 17-year-old son too. This could be my child." This is all I ever wanted, was for someone to care enough to try. I knew there were no certainties, but my son's life was defiantly worth a try. If I could have given my liver to my son for him to live, I would have bided this world a farewell. God's ways are not like ours.

It was now *time for surgery*. October 17, 2013, we arrived at Methodist University on Union at 6:00 AM. I was prayed up, therefore, I had absolutely no worries that my son wouldn't have a successful surgery. I wanted my son to live, and that was my main concern. There are several myths concerning **cancer**, but I had to hold fast on what I knew was right for my child. **cancer** will spread if it is exposed to air, is the number one myth that a countless number of individuals believe. This never crossed my mind, but it was on the heart of my cousin. My only thought was, if it wasn't removed, it would worsen and my son would die.

Before the surgery, Dr. Denali met with us in the hallway, and he prayed for my son. This touched my heart and gave me instant chills. I knew for sure that God was in the mist of us. God positioned the right people in my life at the right time.

Ja'Marcus was in surgery for 10 ½ hours, so it was obvious why I had to take two Hydroxyzine. I prayed that the surgeons would be successful at destroying all the **cancer** from my son's abdomen. For that reason, one thing was on my mind. Hypothermic Intraperitoneal Chemotherapy/ HIPEC or hot chemo bath. This is a method of chemotherapy used during surgery to kill **cancer** cells that are not visible. Ja'Marcus would only get the HIPEC if Dr. Denali and his partner were able to remove all cancerous tumors that were visible. After which a heated sterilized chemo solution would be circulated throughout his abdomen for 90 minutes then he would be sewn up.

The hospital's lobby was filled with love and support. My daughter Deshambra, and my sons Chinney and Tra along with my brother and his wife Darlisha, my sister in Christ Erricka my cousin Debra and her children, Willie, Danielle, and Erin were all there sending prayers to heaven on me and my son's behalf. The prayers were working, because I was at total peace. Having a great support system was a blessing. They were very helpful during this time. No words were needed, just their presence made me happy.

I was in a light sleep when I heard my phone rang. It was Dr. Denali.

I was anxious to know what he had to say, so I quickly answered my phone with a faint hello. "We were able to remove all the cancerous tumors from your son's abdomen, diaphragm, spleen, and intestine." We are about to apply the HIPEC. He is doing well. I will call you back once the surgery is completed" he said. Everyone in the lobby was starting at me with a nervous look and wondering what the doctor had said. I was very emotional, so I simply nodded my head to them, and gave a thumb up. Everyone began embracing one another and praising God. My child had a second chance at life.

Hours after talking to Dr. Denali on the phone, he finally walked off the elevator to the lobby where we were waiting. Everyone walked towards him, greeted and thanked him for all he'd done for Ja'Marcus. He gave me a quick, but detailed update on Ja'Marcus' post-surgery condition. "He will have a long healing process. This surgery was very risky, but since he is young, he will be okay" he boldly stated. Hearing this was a huge relief. I thanked Dr. Denali, and he left.

My son was in ICU after surgery, and he seemed to be progressing well. Things were finally fallen in place. Prayers were bombarding heaven on his behalf daily. I felt compelled to stay by his side. ICU has a strict policy concerning individuals staying with patients. I completely ignored their policy. I sent to the cafeteria for food and I used the chair as a bed. My feet would be swollen, but I was not concerned about me. It was all about my son.

Until Jermaine went to get some fresh air one evening and noticed a family in the hallway frantically crying. I walked to where they were, grabbed their hands, and prayed for them. Their mother was slowly passing away. I told them my story, and they were confused. How could I console them, and my son was ill lying in a hospital bed? I was just as puzzled as they were. Where did this part of me come from? I didn't understand. For one, I am an introvert. I am slow to communicate with people. God altered my heart. He took me out of my comfort zone. He was using me. The pieces were slowly coming together, and I was understanding my storm.

"Trust God's process."

The Road to Recovery
Chapter 21

There would be several bumps in *the road to recovery*. Ja'Marcus had been cut vertically down his belly. A few weeks after the surgery, he was given steroids. This caused the wound to heal slowly. He had no appetite, which is extremely essential to the healing process. The stiches started to loosen, causing the wound to reopen. Consequently, a machine known as a wound vac (vacuum assisted closure) had to be used to promote healthy healing. A wound vac decreases the amount of time it takes to heal in addition to lessening the chance of infections and other problems.

This was a major surgery, and it came with a lot of complications that neither one of us were prepared for. For the surgery to go according to plan, Ja'Marcus had to have a colostomy. A colostomy is a surgical technique used to produce an opening for feces and urine to be discharged from the body. He too had a liver resection, where half of his liver was removed. After complaining of pain and numbness in his feet. It was believed he had developed peripheral neuropathy due to the surgery. Peripheral neuropathy is the effect of impairment to the peripheral nerve. It produces chronic pain, numbness, and weakness in the hand and feet. Dr. Denali believed a nerve may have been slightly touched in his belly, and it affected his hands and feet.

Before we left the hospital, I was taught how to look after the wound and properly put on the colostomy bag. I never thought I would be playing a "nurse" to my child. Everything I was taught was very helpful to me. I wanted to take care of my son, not only because he was very particular about others taking care of him, but because it was my responsibility.

After being in the hospital nearly a month, he was discharged. I took him to Dr. Denali's clinic the following week for a check-up. I signed him in and told the nurse immediately he was running a low-grade temperature. She took one look at him, and said "he isn't feeling well." She called us to triage without delay. She informed Dr. Denali Ja'Marcus appeared to be sick. He came in, took one look at him and immediately ordered me to take him back to Methodist University.

His room was prepared when we arrived, and the nurse immediately began taking care of him. God continued to surround us with caring people, since his nurse was heaven sent. She checked on him around the clock. His temperature would not break and this became her primary concern. Blood cultures were taken from his

PICC and double Hickman lines to check for infections. One culture came back with bacteria in the line. The nurse did not label the bottles beforehand, consequently, he underwent another surgery to have both the PICC and double Hickman line removed.

After the surgery, he continued to be monitored carefully. His nurse was convinced that something more serious than the lines were going on. She told me she believed he had septicemia or sepsis. Sepsis occurs when there is a wound or other area of the body develops an infection. This is a life threating condition. "I have to speak with his doctor right away. His temperature will not break and I do not feel comfortable taking care of him anymore. He should be admitted to ICU immediately. If the doctor comes in before I get back tell him I need to speak with him right away" she said nervously, as she closed the door and proceed to walked down the hallway to get his chart. A few seconds later, Dr. Denali knocked at the door. He walked in and the nurse was with him. She explained what Ja'Marcus' symptoms were and he sent him back to ICU within the hour.

Ja'Marcus was sicker than I imagined. He was intubated and put in a medically induced coma. His temperature continued to rise but he could not have any medications for fever. The nurse wanted to give him a dose of Tylenol per the on-call doctor's order, but I would not allow her to do so. Most medications go through the liver, and my son's liver was in no condition to be stressed. Upon telling her this, she looked at me as if I had spoken in another tongue. Ja'Marcus' doctors at St. Jude had taught me well. Blood work was done months after we were admitted to St. Jude to determine what medications was suitable for him, and Tylenol was a medication he could consume. The nurse became upset when I told her he was not taking the Tylenol because it goes primarily through the liver. "The on-call doctor said he would be fine. I am not giving him a full dose" she said in a rather loud tone. "No, he cannot take Tylenol!" I said also in a louder tone. At this point she is furious. She gathers her belongings and starts to walk out, therefore I opened the door for her. Her conduct was unprofessional and it was intolerable. I did not hesitate to buzz the nurse's station for the charge nurse to report her behavior. I immediately requested a new nurse because I was dealing with too much to entertain negativity. I wanted someone who would help my son and I, not cause us more distress. My child was on his death bed. The charge nurse immediately came to our room with an ice filled basin and multiple towels, just as I'd requested. She understood me. She helped me put the cold towels on Ja'Marcus to bring down his temperature. An hour later the fever started to dwindle. She sympathized with me and she understood my level of frustration and she apologized for the previous nurse's behavior.

I may have been labeled as the mother from hell, but this was my child. It was my job to ensure that he was treated with dignity and respect. I refused to allow anyone to come in and disturb his peace of mind. **Cancer** had already invaded his life. No human was going to take away his peace. It was my job to take care of him and I was going to do that by any means necessary.

A few week later, after multiple rounds of antibiotics Ja'Marcus was feeling better. He was taken out of the coma and showed great signs of improvement. Later that week we were finally being cleared to leave Methodist University, and we couldn't have been any happier. We were St. Jude bound!

"Peace enters your heart; the moment God enters your life."

Part III

Back to St. Jude
Chapter 22

On November 20, 2013, we were discharged from Methodist University permanently. We were finally heading **back to St. Jude**. Although he was discharged, he was not well enough to go home, instead we resided at the Ronald McDonald House until one day before Christmas. Ja'Marcus was so pleased to be back in the care of Dr. Freeman, Dr. Elise, and the St. Jude team it brought him to tears. Tears of joy flowed down his cheeks as we walked through the doors. He believed no other doctor understood him as well as Dr. Freeman and Elise. He had gotten use to the them and no one did anything right except St. Jude in his eyes. I was more than thankful since St. Jude knew more about him as a person than any other hospital. His diagnosis was most important, but understanding the whole person is important to me as well.

Ja'Marcus was continuing to heal from the HIPEC surgery. Cleaning and caring for the wound was essential to healing, but taking the dressing off was tremendously painful. Dr. Elise agreed that pulling bandages off the area was not a wise choice. Since the area had to be monitored closely, she thought putting him under to do the procedure would be best. She communicated with Dr. Freeman concerning the matter and he agreed with her. He was sedated with Propofol to change the dressing. This method was very beneficial for he did not have to endure any extra pain. Just watching the doctors at Methodist remove the sticky bandages from his skin, right where he'd been cut was devastating for us both. The wound care nurse always did a good job with dressing the wound. She took pictures of his healing process. She thought using a wound vac would better help him to heal. A wound vac (vacuum assisted closure) is a machine used to remove blood and other fluids from an operational site or wound. Using this device helps the wound to heal better and quicker. He continued to use the wound vac for nearly six weeks. Once the wound had healed, we celebrated him being one month free of abdominal **cancer**. The look on his face will leave an everlasting impression on my heart. Knowing the **cancer** was gone, happy is a mere understatement. There is no word to describe how he felt about God given him a second chance at life.

  Ja'Marcus started having issues walking and holding things in his hand a few weeks after the surgery. I was originally told at Methodist University he had developed peripheral neuropathy, but it was not diagnosed. I discussed my concerns about the "peripheral neuropathy" with Dr. Elise. All the symptoms he displayed, led her to believe he may have had peripheral neuropathy as well. The pain was unrelenting; so, she wrote him a prescription for pain medication with hopes this would help to ease the pain. Unfortunately, the pain medication was not successful. The pain seemed to worsen. She considered during a spinal tap, to determine if there was another under lying problem, and it was. After getting the spinal tap results back, he was diagnosed with Guillain-Barre Syndrome. Guillain-Barre Syndrome is a rare illness, where the body's immune system attacks the nerves. Now that we had a diagnosis, he was given the proper medication to treat the issue. Although the medication did not stop the pain, it gave him a quality of life.

Now that the big surgery was completed, it was now time to focus on the small masses on his lungs. CT scans were done to confirm the **cancer** was stable. It had not grown since March 2013. Dr. Elise and Freeman looked over the scans, and explained it was not a good idea to put his body through another stressful surgery too soon. His body needed to get stronger before considering another surgical procedure. The mass would be monitored periodically for any significant alterations.

> **"And call upon me in the day of trouble: I will deliver thee, and thou shalt glorify me."**
>
> **Psalm 50:15 (KJV)**

Lord, Not Again

Chapter 23

Ja'Marcus found it to be more comfortable sleeping in Big Mama's recliner after his surgery. The end of April 2014, he began complaining of stomach pain. "It is back" I thought after examining the area of the pain. I felt something, but I did not let him know that I believed it was a mass. I knew in his mind he knew that the **cancer** had come back, therefore, we went to God in prayer.

We were heading to St. Jude in a few days, so I decided to wait until his appointment to tell his doctor about the mass. Once we made it to the hospital, I told Dr. Elise about the pain and the area of the pain. She immediately ordered for him to have a full body CT scan. The results came back, the **cancer** had returned. "***Lord, not again!***" I said as I felled to the floor in tears. We were destroyed. It was unbearable to see the hurt on his face. "Stop crying. I am going to be okay" he said. I wanted to stop, but the tears kept rolling down my face. The last thing I want was for my son to die. I didn't want to imagine life without my child. I was destroyed by the thoughts.

The only option I had was prayer.

We would travel to St. Jude Children's Research Hospital for treatments every two weeks. He was now on a clinical trial chemo drugs. This chemotherapy treatment was not as severe as the first round of chemo. There were no major side effects and this time, he did not lose his hair. We continued to pray with hopes this treatment would kill the **cancer** cells. We knew there were no guarantees, but hope was all we had to hold on to.

Jesus did not promise us an easy life. John 16:33 says the opposite; "I have told you these things, so that in me you may have peace in this world you will have trouble. But take heart! I have overcome the world." This is proof that trials and tribulations are not by accident. We must trust that in the middle of the storm God is already there. We must go through the storm and learn to fully rely on Him. Treading through the storm helped me to build my faith. Without storms, one will never know how strong they are. I've oftentimes said, "I wouldn't know what to do if one of my children died." Life would be pointless, instead life goes on.

... weeping may endure for a night, but joy cometh in the morning

0Psalm 30:5 (KJV)

Trouble Doesn't Last Always
Chapter 24

Big Mama use to say, *"**trouble doesn't last always**"*, so we held onto the belief that God was going to heal him, therefore we prayed every day for a miracle that could only be explained by God. At times, I felt as if God had forgotten about me because I was not ready to answer this question. I was floored with a decision that I knew someday would come. "If your son passes away do you want him to be resuscitated?" Dr. Elise asked me. I stared at her as if she'd asked the craziest question I had ever heard. She caught me totally off guard, and I quickly changed the subject. I was thinking, "yes, I want you to do whatever you have been trained to do to save a human life. If my son stops breathing, you better make him breath again." Just the thoughts of my son dying, brought me to tears. She'd asked me this question multiple times and frankly, I was sick of it. I decided to talk to Ja'Marcus' medication nurse about this resuscitating situation. She ensured me she would talk to Dr. Elise about the matter. I did not want her to ask me about this again. I knew it was important that she knew, but I was not mentally ready to deal it. When I was ready to talk about it, she'd be the first to know.

I'd put the conversation off long enough, but it was important I knew what my son wanted. This was his life and he deserved to make his own decisions. During a casual conversation between my son and I, I asked him if he wanted to be resuscitated when he passed away. He did not fully understand what resuscitating meant. I explained to him what occurs when one must be resuscitated. His exact words were, "if I pass away, apparently it is my time to go. Let me go." BOOM! I was flabbergasted! It was like a bomb had exploded in our den. I did not expect my 18-year-old son to express himself with such boldness. His answer is what my soul needed to calm my fears of him dying. A few months after Ja'Marcus' diagnosis, we had a conversation that I would never forget. He stood in the den with his eyes full of tears and he uttered, "I love you so much momma. I don't want to die and leave you." With a convincing and bold tone, I

Death is a topic that is rarely discussed, but it is a vital part of life. It was important that Dr. Elise knew what he wanted, but it was more important that I knew. May 2, 2014 was the day I signed the papers for my son to die a natural death. She was stunned when I told her Ja'Marcus' wishes. "I know this was difficult for you both, but it is something that we need to know, just in case it happens suddenly" she said. Some days the storm gave me the impression it would never cease. I was being knocked down constantly from the force of the strong winds. Everyday brought something new except a rainbow, but I never took my focus off God. I held His hand during the storm, because one day, someday, the sun will shine again.

"The strongest people find faith and courage during a storm."

Another Bump in the Road
Chapter 25

I was cooking one evening, when Ja'Marcus asked me to change is colostomy bag. I could tell from where he was looking he wasn't looking at the colostomy. I walked to his recliner, and noticed he had two small holes in his abdomen that were directly on the surgical incision. I was scared out of my mind. "Where did these holes come from. Was the **cancer** eating through his flesh" I said out loud. I didn't know if I should move him, so I called 911. When they arrived, they immediately bombarded me what seemed like 21 questions in less than a minute. No sir! I was in no mood for answering questions. They only thing that I needed to do was to get my son to the emergency room without delay. I asked the quiet paramedic to please move the ambulance, as I was about to drive my son to the hospital myself. My husband picked Ja'Marcus up from his recliner, put him the truck, and we headed to the emergency room. This was the day I learned, NEVER to call 911 in an emergency.

Before any procedures were done, the ER doctor would call St.

Jude beforehand, since this was St. Jude's protocol. The local hospital always went above and beyond for my son. With every visit, the staff had a caring spirit and was eager to help. This made my heart glad. The last thing a caregiver should be concerned about is one being rude to their love one. I believe medical professionals must have a genuine love for the care and well-being of the patient, and North Sunflower Medical Center displayed this affection.

I explained in full details the type of **cancer** that my son had, how the **cancer** developed, the type of surgery he had and the severity of the surgery. The ER doctor had heard of the HIPEC surgery, but never met an individual that had the procedure done. He was absolutely bewildered, and had no clue what could have caused the open wounds on Ja'Marcus' belly. Nevertheless, he was very concerned and began asking questions concerning his health before the **cancer**. He was in complete awe that I knew as much as I did about my son's diagnosis. "Most parents come in and only know the shape and color of the medication" he stated. That was not an option for me. My son needed me. Therefore, I had to educate myself fully on his **cancer**, the cause of his **cancer**, every medication that he is prescribed, and each procedure that he has.

The opened area continued to ooze a brownish fluid that carried an odd smell. At this point, the goal was to hurriedly clean and cover the opened wound to reduce his chances of getting an infection. Per the doctor's order, the nurse cleaned and placed a colostomy bag over the area. After he spoke with the on-call doctor at St. Jude, I was informed to take him to St. Jude the following day to see his oncologists.

Before going to Memphis, I called Dr. Elise and gave her the details of what happened the previous night and what was going on now. She wanted me to bring him to the hospital right away. When we arrived, she and her medical team were waiting on our arrival, and we were seen immediately. With just one look, we had a clear diagnosis, but the prognosis wasn't what neither of us wanted to hear. Ja'Marcus had developed a gastrointestinal fistula. A gastrointestinal fistula is an uncommon opening in one's stomach. This opening causes intestinal fluids to leak through the lining of the intestine or abdomen. A person that has a tumor or **cancer** is more likely to develop a fistula. In Ja'Marcus' case, his skin was very thin, due to the HIPEC surgery. The thin layer of skin made him more prone to develop a gastrointestinal fistula. I administered antibiotics to him daily. He was now wearing two colostomy bags, and Dr. Elise believed he'd be wearing the second one indefinitely. The chances of the fistula closing were slim to none. The brownish fluid was defection, which naturally contains a countless number of bacteria, which is not healthy. This is especially true for **cancer** patients. For this reason, we began entering the hospital from the back at the Ambulatory Care Unit (ACU) or Isolation. We followed this procedure with every visit to keep other patient's free of germs. We'd come to ***another bump in the road***, but it was nothing prayer would not fix.

"Pray and trust God's timing."

Lifetime of Memories
Chapter 26

Some days the storm gave me the impression it would never cease. I felt as if I was being knocked down repeatedly from the energy of the potent winds. In my hours of weakness, I kneeled to Him in prayer. For everyday seemed to bring something new, except a rainbow. There were days the devil tried to creep in, but I never took my heart off God and His word. I held His hand tighter since I knew God was the head of my ship. One day, someday, the sun will shine again. But when? God was molding me into the person He knew I could be. He did not place me in the ship to set sail alone or to weather the storm in vain. There were things I needed to learn alone; just God and me. This could only be accomplished by me learning how to survive in the storm.

As Ja'Marcus health continued to deteriorate, a part of me began to fade. It tore me up inside to watch him wither away right before my eyes. We continued our weekly doctor visits, and he continued to take Sorafenib daily to keep the **cancer** stable. I had come to the realization, there was nothing more that could be done to cure my son. The HIPEC was successful, but the **cancer** refused to leave my son alone. It was now I recalled the doctor's words from Jackson concerning the Sorafenib. I prayed to God more than ever that He would spare my firstborn's life. I prayed that my child be healed, but when the c word came back it came with a vengeance. It had ruined my child's physical body. The masses in his stomach began to spread like wildfire and the spots on his lungs had gotten bigger. He had been given a Morphine filled pain pump to keep his pain at bay. This helped him to live comfortably.

While the **cancer** was growing, my faith was too. The Lord had not brought me this far to watch me drown. I watched my son take his first breath and I was preparing to watch him take his final breath. I was mentally arranging my son's funeral. Who will he be buried by? What color will his casket be? What will he wear? Where will the funeral be held? These were the questions I asked myself as I walked to the kitchen table with my pen and pad.

Despite the growing **cancer**, the fistula, and the colostomy, Ja'Marcus made the best of each day. His pain level was zero to nonexciting. He now had enough strength to go outside and enjoy life. Church meant everything to him and he missed going. He was in no condition to attend church every Sunday since his walking had decreased tremendously. There were days that he felt great, and I would take him to church. I would push him to the front of the church since this is where he'd normally sit. I could tell by the look on his face that worship was what his heart needed. Attending church would be the highlight of his day. He would often tell me he was going to lead songs again, but he did not have enough strength to lead songs again. If he felt well enough to sing, he would have. I knew God understood this and this gave us both peace. He loved guns, but I trusted him with only B.B. guns. I would take him outside occasionally to shoot at the target his step-father had made and attached to the tree. Since he had to sit in his wheelchair, to keep him from feeling odd, we all sat down. I wanted him to enjoy life as much as possible. This gave him a magnificent sense of "being normal."

Ja'Marcus and I started taking random pictures every day. We were making a lifetime of memories. Regardless of what happened, I would have a collection of happy and sad times. Making a ***lifetime of memories***, by capturing every sweet moment with my son would be a joyful blessing to me. With each photograph, we smiled as if it was our last portrait together. Our conversations were full of fun and laughter, even when our hearts were filled with tears of sorrow. Many deemed it ironic since they could not understand how we had joy when our world was crumbling. The unspeakable joy that flowed through our souls came from on high. A fresh dose of God's peace filled our hearts day-to-day.

-When someone you love becomes a memory...that memory becomes a treasure.

The End Was Nearing

Chapter 27

Ja'Marcus' siblings would come to his room each morning before leaving for school to check on him. They would chat for a while and they would say their good-byes. This morning was no different, but there was a slight twist. At 7:15 my son had a voice, and at 8:00 it was gone. He'd went from talking to simply staring in the matter of minutes.

Months after being discharged from the hospital, Ja'Marcus fell into another lethargic state. I initially thought his ammonia level had increased, so I contacted Dr. Elise. Since he was not sleeping excessively, an elevated ammonia level was ruled out. She ordered me to continue to monitor him, and I did so for three days. He still wasn't responding, but he'd move his head and smile when I asked him a question. I started to panic and needed to know why he was sluggish. For this reason, I called Dr. Elise, and voiced my concerns to her. She quickly stated, "Take him to the local ER." Within the hour, my husband and I dressed and took him to the hospital.

Everyone knew Ja'Marcus' condition at Ruleville Medical Center. Once we arrived, we were taken to triage immediately. He was instantly given oxygen to help him breath, since his level was low. The ER doctor thought it would help him better if he monitored Ja'Marcus' condition throughout the day. After several hours of being observed, the doctor could not determine what was happening. He contacted St. Jude and an ambulance traveled from Memphis to transport my son and I to St. Jude.

On October 21, 2014, I walked into the hallways of St. Jude once again. Hope goes before me with each hospital visit, but somehow this visit felt unusual. I was awfully anxious. Walking into the unknown is heart-wreaking. I've witness my son go inside this hospital several times and beat the odds by walking out. I fervently bombarded heaven's door with prayers of hope that my son would come home.

Dr. Elise greeted us at the back entrance of the hospital. A triage nurse was with her, and she quickly took Ja'Marcus' vitals and escorted us to his assigned room. Each medication that triggered drowsiness was stopped and the Morphine was decreased. Dr. Freeman and Elise ensured he was being monitored carefully. During this hospital stay, I did not stay. My brother Tradanius and sister Soprina gave me a break. They took turns spending the night with him.

If there was an emergency Dr. Elise would call me. When the doctor and nurses would come to the room to check on him or to administer medication, my siblings would FaceTime or text me. I was being updated as if I was there.

I was thankful for my brother and sister because my middle daughter began having mental problems that started January 2014. I'd scheduled appointments for her to see multiple psychiatrists and I needed to be at home to take her to her doctor visits, for parental support, and I needed to spend time with my other children. Everyone was dealing with Ja'Marcus' illness in a different way and simply being with them comforted each of us.

On October 26, I received a call from Ja'Marcus' quality of life nurse. She gave me the latest update on his condition, which was basically the same in addition to asking when was I coming to the hospital. Once she asked this question, I knew something more serious was going on; more than she'd told me. "I'll be there tomorrow morning as soon as I take my children to school" I softly spoke. "Great, I will see you then" she uttered in an optimistic tone. I immediately began praying. The last thing I wanted to hear was bad news, but somehow, I knew bad news was in the making.

The next morning, my drive to St. Jude was optimistic. I had to remain positive although the devil was trying to get the best of me.

This drive alone gave me a chance to truly pray and meditate on God's word thorough spiritual acapella music. This had been a long journey, but God has been faithful. He's been with me through the good times and the bad. If He allowed me to make it this far, I knew I could continue without unwavering faith. It normally takes me 2 hours to drive to Memphis, but today was different. I arrived at the hospital in one hour and 30 minutes. Time was of the essence and I was in dire need to know why I it was urgent for me to come to the hospital. Once again, I was pacing into uncertainties. Entering a world of unknowns is petrifying. As I walked to my son's room, I could hear my heartbeat. With each step, I wanted to turn around and run the other direction, but I continued to walk by faith. I knew there was a higher force because the human side of me could not have done it. There is a God.

    I stood quietly outside of my son's room. I prayed then I walked in. I went straight to his bedside grabbed him by the hand and kissed his forehead. He opened his eyes and looked at me as I talked to him, but he didn't say a word. Shortly after my arrival, his medical team knocked and entered the room. I could tell by the look on their faces something was horribly wrong. They greeted me with a gloomy hello and immediately asked me to walk to the parent room which was next door to Ja'Marcus' room.

    "Ja'Marcus has been here 6 days. We have taken him off all medications that may possibly cause him to be drowsy. His pain medication causes drowsiness, but we decreased it as much as possible, but he's still lethargic and no medicine is causing it. You are a great mother. You're one of the best mothers I have seen. You're always so organized and prepared. You were right by your son's side every step of the way. You've had to make decisions that were hard, but you did it. We've seen you laugh and cry. Ja'Marcus has been an amazing patient. He's brighten my day on many occasions. It's been a real pleasure knowing him and being his provider. It breaks my heart to tell you this, but he is transitioning. There is nothing more we at St. Jude can do for him. Do you want him to stay here to be monitored around the clock or do you want to take him home?" the nurse softly said. I put my face in my hand and I sobbed. I cried not for my son, but for me. I'd never been so heartbroken. I'd heard of others being told "there is nothing more we can do for you", but now I was experiencing it. This is worse than hearing your son has cancer. It appeared that everything was happening so quickly. I soon gathered my composure and with a shaky voice uttered, "he is going home. Thank you all for all you've done for my son and me. We were blessed to have such a caring medical team." I sobbed as I signed the discharge papers.

The storm had gotten stronger, but this was only an opening for my prayers to go higher. Even in the middle of the sea God is still there and He is in full control. He governs the final say over life and death. He gave it and only He can take it.

I walked back to my son's room, looked at him, went inside the bathroom and broke down weeping. My heart was totally shattered. The first person that I knew loved me unconditionally was slowly physically leaving me. My mind begins racing with thoughts. How am I going to live without my son? How am I going to tell my children their big brother is about to die? Lord are you going to put me through this again? I know God can do anything but fail! Please Lord intervene and let my son live. I would do anything for him to live! I was begging God to not take my boy away from me. Okay Lord at this point, it is fine if he lives with **cancer**. I will continue to be there and take care of him. I will endure with every struggle that is thrown my way, just let my son live.

How selfish of me! Everything I was thinking was for my own satisfaction. I honestly wanted my child to live, but if **cancer** had to be a part of him I'd let him go. The hardest decision I ever had to make was to prepare to say "good-bye" to my son, so I didn't. ***The end was nearing*** on earth, but we will meet again. I have no doubts.

For to me to live is Christ, and to die is gain. If I am to live in the flesh, that means fruitful labor for me. Yet which I shall choose I cannot tell. I am hard pressed between the two. My desire is to depart and be with Christ, for that is far better.

Philippians 1:21-23

The Physical Journey Home
Chapter 28

The physical journey home was October 27th which is Ja'Marcus' baby brother's birthday. My son arrived from St. Jude Children's Research Hospital by ambulance and I was excited he was finally home. I was standing at the door waiting on their arrival and to greet him with open arms. The paramedics slowly backed into the driveway, opened the doors, walked to the back of the ambulance, pulled Ja'Marcus' gurney out and proceeded to bring him in the house. They were generous enough to transport him to his room and position him in the bed. As they prepared to leave, one of the paramedics expressed his compassion by saying "we are praying for Ja'Marcus. We hope he pulls through. He is a good kid, so I've heard. I will pray for him." I smiled, nodded and with a gentle "thank-you" I extended my hand to shake their hand for all they'd done. I am always grateful for amazing healthcare professionals.

I was given clear details on how to care for him. His body had become extremely tender to touch, so I limited full bed baths to simple sponge baths. Since he was lethargic, he could not eat, but I continued to give him the total parenteral nutrition or TPN. The TPN was his primary source of nutrition which was administered intravenously. The TPN supplied him with nutrients such as lipids, amino acids, glucose, salts, dietary minerals, and added vitamins.

` I was given peppermint sponges from the hospital to clean his mouth because he couldn't brush his teeth. I thought it was convenient since I knew he'd like to taste something besides water. I would dip the sponge in orange, apple, or grape juice and he'd suck the juice out of the sponge. The thoughts of him missing out on life hurt my spirit more than anything so I tried to keep things as normal as possible. We'd prayed the **cancer** would go away and he would return to be a normal teenager. I guess God had other plans. We could only do what he allowed, therefore, we played the cards we were dealt the best way we knew how.

Family Feud was Ja'Marcus' favorite game show. He and I would pick a family to be and compete with one another. At 9:00 every morning I would turn to Family Feud and although he wasn't talking, I knew he could hear me talk to him. I would ask him which team he wanted to be and assumed he was okay with it. After days of not talking or even mumbling, one morning we were watching Family Feud. My team was winning of course, and I said, "Ja'Marcus your team is sorry" and out of the blue he mumbled something. I turned around in complete shock and said loudly, "are you trying to tell me something" and he nodded his head "yes" with a faint but noticeable and beautiful smile. I hadn't seen my son smile in weeks. You can only imagine how I felt.

There's this saying, "when an ill person stops talking and suddenly starts back, they are getting better to die." I thought this was the most insane thing I'd ever heard *but keep reading*. Days passed and there was no change, until nearly the end of his first week back home. I was turning the T.V. to Family Feud after giving him a bath and clothing him when he said, "I sure could eat me a big breakfast mommy." I dropped the remote in amazement since this voice came out of nowhere. It was a blessing for me to hear his voice once again. After thanking God, I answered him, "What do you want to eat. You can't swallow hard foods." Without a second thought he said, "bacon, eggs, grits, and toast." I used my better judgement and cooked him grits and soft scrambled eggs. I hurried and cooked his food. I was so ready to see him eat. I walked to his room with his favorite breakfast food and I fed him. He was ready to eat because he consumed everything. He was able drink his juice from a cup with no complications. There was no greater joy for me this day.

The children came home from school, walked to the room to speak to Ja'Marcus and he said "hey!" After the quick "hey", he began saying complete sentences that everyone in the house heard and understood. The kids were shocked. Everyone began laughing and talking. It truly felt like old times. He loved his iPhone, therefore, his next sentences were "Where is my phone? Give it to me." Without delay, I handed him the phone. Later in the day, he called everyone's name in the house, but he was looking for one person. He couldn't seem to get the name out, then he finally articulated "Where is Jermaine? Can ya'll get Jermaine for me?" Everyone but my aunt and I left the room. The children were running to get my husband. My husband and Ja'Marcus had a special bond. He looked for Jermaine to be there to help him maneuver around without a lot of hassle, and he was always right there. Although Jermaine was not Ja'Marcus' biological father, he helped me to care for him from the beginning to the end.

Ja'Marcus continued to talk for a few more days. God had heard my prayers and I was certain my son was going to defy the doctor's prognosis. One cold cloudy evening his cousin came by to visit him. It appeared as if he was attempting to fall back into the lethargic state, but when I asked him did he know the young man standing before him, he looked, nodded and said, "That is Deon. What's up man? I want some chicken. Will you go to Church's and get me some?" Deon was not in a car, but he walked to the store in what seemed like 5 minutes. Once he came back to the house and walked in the room with the food, Ja'Marcus had went back into the lethargic state. 5 minutes is all it took for things to take another awful detour.

I'd noticed that he was not urinating as much as he should, but he wasn't consuming a lot of food or liquid either. Normally when his stoma is stimulated or if it was uncovered for a while, it would produce stool, but this was not happening. A stoma is an artificial opening on the wall of one's abdomen to collect waste. The stoma may be temporary or permanent, but in Ja'Marcus' situation, the stoma was permanent.

I bathed him and changed his colostomy bag to see and measure how much he was putting out. The entire day passed and there was nothing. I began to grow concern because I knew this meant his kidneys were not functioning properly. Throughout his diagnosis, his eyes remained white, until now. Jaundice had now developed. His eyes were dark yellow and he simply look as if he was staring into space.

St. Jude connected us with a local hospice agency. His nurse was more than helpful to us. She came out to visit on her scheduled days and she ensured Ja'Marcus' received top quality care. Before we used Sunflower Hospice, we used another agency and the service that the nurses provided were horrible. I was glad Ruleville had a quality hospice agency, because the nurse Ja'Marcus had was simply the best nurse in the Mississippi Delta. I've seen several nurses that are nurses for the money, but not this nurse. She went above and beyond to ensure that Ja'Marcus was happy, relax, and comfortable always. Whatever he wanted or needed, you can guarantee Ms. Jenette Watson was going to get it. He loved green Powerade, and she purchased them almost daily for whom she called "her boy."

She was nothing short of astounding. Words cannot express my gratitude towards her. I trusted her judgment in all things since she'd shown me her genuine care for her patients. Although Ms. Watson wasn't Ja'Marcus' current nurse, I continued to call her for answers to my questions.

That old saying "when an ill person stops talking and suddenly starts back, they are getting better to die", I learned this saying was true. I prepared and feed my son his last meal just as I did his first. I was now ready for God to do what He saw fit.

"God has a reason for allowing things to happen. We may never understand His wisdom, but we must trust His will."

I am Next

Chapter 29

When Aunt Shirley passed away, our hearts were destroyed for she was one of the primary pillars of our family. I was torn inwardly. She was my physical guiding light during my son's illness. She helped me more than she knew, and know she was gone. "We live to die" is what she would often say, therefore, I knew that she did not want me to mourn her death. Her focus was for me to take care of my son. I wanted to protect Ja'Marcus. I did not want to hurt him by telling him Aunt Shirley had passed away. I knew the anguish of this news would be a great burden on him, but like always he was fine.

Big Mama had taken ill and was admitted into the hospital for several months. Everyone went about their daily lives, because this wasn't the first time she'd been admitted into the hospital. She did not appear to be dreadfully ill, but she was. We were at St. Jude Children's Research Hospital when I learned that my Big Mama had passed. I was dazed! Moving away from Ruleville was never an option when my granny was alive, since I wanted to be by her side when she took her final breathe. Now look at my situation! I was two hours away from her. I wanted to be there, but she knew I had to take care of my son. I begged my Aunt Margaret to tell the mortician not to take her away until I made it home. The speed limit was 65, but I did 80 until I made it to the woman who raised me.

When I arrived at the house, the mortician was driving up. I jumped out of the truck and rushed to my granny's bedside. I was shocked at what I observed. Her face looked as if she had put on her mocha powder. "Who put makeup on her" I asked as I smiled, sobbed, and kissed her flawless skin. My aunt sadly replied, "she doesn't have on makeup." I could not believe my eyes, she was absolutely beautiful. Aunt Shirley was assuredly the rock in our family, but Big Mama was the head cornerstone. What was our family going to do now? We all were at a complete loss, and all we could do was pray. This was the second immediate death in our family, but God makes no errors.

Later in the day, Ja'Marcus and his siblings sat in the den and talked amongst themselves. "*I am next*. Don't tell momma. I don't want her to be upset, but I am going to die next" were the words I was later told he said. "Chinney, I need you to look out for the kids; especially our baby sister Skylar. They are going to need you. You are going to be the oldest when I leave. Don't cry for me. You all will have to be strong for momma" he told them. Ja'Marcus wanted his younger brother, Chinney to be prepared to take on the big brother role. He was strong and he wanted his brothers and sisters to be strong as well. When my children told me what Ja'Marcus had told them I was speechless. I used to hear my grandmother say, an ill person feels their death approaching. I don't know if this is true, but by the words my son spoke, made me wonder; did he feel his time was nearing? I knew at this point, I had given birth to my hero.

"This world is not my home. I'm just passing through."

His Final Breath
Chapter 30

As the week continued Ja'Marcus slept in complete silence. I continued to give him sponge baths, cleaned his mouth, and ensured he was comfortable. Not knowing whether he was in pain, I continued to give boluses of Morphine throughout the day. Being by my son's side was important to me. I was obligated to be right there, therefore, I sat and slept by his bedside 24-7, only getting up to use the bathroom.

November 13, 2014 is when things started to dwindle and fast. Around 4:30 Ms. Jeanette came by to check on him. I suspected that he was slowly drifting away, but I wanted to be certain. I asked her to go into the room and look at him. Upon doing so, she dropped her head, walked down the hallway and nodded "yes." "Are you going to call his nurse?" she asked. "No ma'am. I want to be the only one with him when he takes his final breath. I will call her afterwards" I sadly stated. I assumed watching my son pass away would be the hardest thing I had to do, but I reminded myself of the year and eight-month storm that we'd sailed. Understanding that I had prayed he'd be healed gave me great relief. Although every part of me wanted him to live and be healed of **cancer**, but in a spiritual sense; death is the ultimate form of healing. God's plans did not align with mine, nevertheless I had confidence that His will was greatly divine.

His father knocked at the door nearly an hour later. Really?!??? This was unquestionably unexpected. The time had come for your son to expire, and you decide to see him? What happened to last week, the previous week, and the weeks before? What could have been more important than trying to be by your **cancer** stricken son's side during this unfortunate tragedy? This is the least he could have done since he wasn't an instrumental part of his life. With these questions running through my mind, I basically opened the door, walked outside and conversed with him about Ja'Marcus' current state. "My son is dying." I miserably murmured. He looked at me, but no words came from his mouth. He was mute. I could see the pain all over his face. Was he hurt because his son was dying or was it guilt? If you instantly thought guilt, you are exactly right. He now feels the wrath of not being a father to his son, even during death. He didn't even ask me if he could see his son for the last time. He was now suffering, but I could not feel sorry for him. I never denied him the opportunity to bond with his child. He chose to not be a part of his son's life. This is a decision that he made and it will forever be embedded within his spirit. After a brief conversation, he left and I went to be by my son's side. While Ja'Marcus' father was a close relative, his demeanor was distance; but

I forgave him.

As time progressed, death was approaching like a thief in the night. I monitored him closely and around 9:30 I began to hear an unusual sound known as the "death rattle." For hours, the rattling was on and off. His breathing became shallow, then regular again. Granting he was asleep, he could still hear me. I continued telling him that I loved him and I needed him to keep praying. For the last time, I asked him if he was in pain, and he nodded "no." Even at the end of my storm, God still found a way to make my heart joyful. It was at this point, I was at complete peace at what God was doing.

Many of you may have seen the video I posted on his Joy4Jay Facebook page. I was telling you that he was fading away without saying the exact word, since I did not want him to hear me and become uneasy. Throughout this time, his breathing had become awfully shallow, but minutes later it regulated. I checked his blood pressure several times, and it was fluctuating. My son was dying to live. He is the definition of fighter. I recalled Christiana telling me she had to tell her son Max it was okay if he left her and she'd be fine. I just couldn't bring myself to say those words, until his breathing continued to alter.

Ja'Marcus and I shared a special bond as mother and son, and it was only far that I allowed him to take his final rest. Again, I'd fell back into my selfish ways, so, I kissed his hand, and expressed myself,

"I love you more than you'll ever know. I will always be your momma. You are a great son, but it is okay if you leave me. I will be just fine." After saying those words, his breathing became shallow again. He continued to breath in this manner until 4:40. The rattling in his throat had ceased. I checked his blood pressure again, since now his breathing was faint. There was barely a rise and fall of his chest. After checking his pressure three times I finally said, "Ja'Marcus, what are you doing? I need a pressure, but please keep talking to God baby." I tried once more to get a pressure but still nothing. I took the cuff from around his arm, after which he took his final breath. The first thing I did when my son succumbed was disconnect the pain pumps. I prayed that my son be healed, and now he was. I was there with him when he took his first and **his final breath**. Eczema, ADHD, and sleep apnea was no competition to **cancer**. Even with the proper treatment, my son surly died.

LOVE NEVER FAILS
I Cor. 13:8

How Bold is Cancer?

Chapter 31

Did you notice that throughout the book, the word **Cancer** is **Bold**? Why? **Cancer boldly** walks in our life and attempts to destroy our temple. It gradually tiptoes in and interrupts our daily living and deprives the body of it's healthy condition. **Cancer** slowly beats down the immune system leaving one tired, sicker, sluggish, a sense of void and oftentimes lifeless. Do you realize there are somethings **cancer** cannot do? **Cancer** is very restricted. It does not have the capability to take away one's belief in Christ. This trust has been implanted by a Higher source. It cannot destroy a person's hope, for confidence is rooted within the heart. **Cancer** is so imperfect. Its voice is crippled by silence, but it cannot silence the voices that speaks out against it. Though **Cancer** steals lives, it does not have the authority to abolish one's inner strength. Inner strength is created by daily supplications unto Christ. **Cancer** is so restrained. It cannot cease one's prayers to heaven. **Cancers** imperfectness truly amazes me. It creeps in with limited power seeking to defeat its opponent. It fails to realize its adversary will gain a crown of righteousness when the storm is over, since **Cancer** cannot defeat a Christian. **Cancer**, do you realize your presence makes one stronger? Yes, you cause unimaginable suffering, but you do not have the ability to take away one's peace of mind. Do you realize you are the reason one's faith is renewed in Christ? Do you understand you cannot destroy anyone, unless their Father in Heaven gives you permission? **Cancer** is not clever. It doesn't realize it can destroy lives, bodies, and change families, but it cannot shatter eternal salvation. Eternal salvation is given by Christ and only He. Our physical body was designed to die, but our spiritual soul shall live again. **Cancer** is bold, it can destroy and kill one's body, however, Jesus is bolder. We can live again, if we only know Him.

My Letter to Cancer

Dear **Cancer**,

I won't pretend I like you. I hate you with every being of my heart. For it is because of you that my son and I are apart. To know my son, is to know his journey. He fought you and God was his army. He was devout, inspirational, smart and humble. His mind stayed on Jesus so he would not stumble. You attacked his life and Christ called him home. This left me broken. My soul crumbled, without him I feel all alone. The Lord is present this I truly know. He reigns on high, this is where my blessings flow. He knows my anguish He knows my pain. Thoughts of living without my son, makes my world seem insane. I hate **Cancer** is what I constantly say. You caused me to miss my son every single day. You are limited. There are things you cannot do. You did not stop me from holding God's hand. For He is who I am conformed too. **Cancer** you are cripple. You should come with a cane. For what God has for my son and I, you cannot detain. You are horrible, vile and mean. But you could not destroy my son's spiritual being. **Cancer**, I have no respect for you and I never will. You took my son's life, but his soul you could not kill.

Signed,

A Blessed Mother In Spite Of Your Existence

The Burial of a Hero
Chapter 32

The day my son died, was the day my soul died. My life will never be the same. I was emotionally suffering, but no tears would flow from my eyes. I promptly recognized even though my son was dead, my soul had been spiritually lifted. No mother of sound mind could possibly be telling others "Ja'Marcus is okay. Wipe those tears away, because he was a Christian." It's unimaginably odd, but I felt my mind was on a higher level. Christ had moved all tears from my heart, now I had the ability to help others. I could not believe my actions, but God works in mysterious ways.

After detaching the pain pumps from his PICC line, I posted "Jayy is an angel now" on his Facebook page. As I typed those words, I felt a great sensation of harmony. This was a form of peace that surpasses all comprehension. Normally my Facebook gets quite at an hour of the night, but on November 13th and early morning 14th 2014, Facebook was active. Once I posted the status, my wall lit up with "I am praying for you" and other encouraging words. I could not believe all the support that my son and I had. I received messages not only from Mississippi, but as far as New York, Georgia, Tennessee and D.C. (just to name a few). Many of these individuals were people that were following Ja'Marcus' Facebook page. The phone calls and text messages were relentless, and I embraced each one. This extra boost of love gave me the zeal to continue to move on. Although there were times I wanted to break down. I needed to scream and cry, but I had so much encouragement and support it was impossible to do so now.

After posting the status, I then calmly walked to the room where my husband was asleep and told him the painful news. I thought telling my children would be the most difficult, but it wasn't. The older children held up rather well, while the younger children were devastated. I could tell Chinney and Deshambra were heartbroken, but they did not show it. I then walked to the laundry room and called the home health to let her know my son had passed away. "I will be there shortly" she stated in a calm tone.

Five minutes after I posted the status on Facebook, my childhood friends, Rita and Tammy were the first ones to knock at my door. I have been friends with these sisters for a lifetime. They referred to my son as being their nephew. I allowed them to come in the room where my son's unresponsive body lied. They were grief-stricken, for they wept as if he was their own. The older children prepared for their day and went to school for they could not deal with the stress of being idle. They were close to Ja'Marcus and once he became ill, their bond heightened to a higher level. This is another time my children experienced hurt and I felt helpless.

This entire process was new but preparing for the funeral wasn't as difficult as I expected it to be. Months before he passed away, I contemplated writing his obituary. I started, but I did not complete it. Now, I was sitting at my kitchen table gathering information and pictures to prepare for *the burial of a hero*. There were times I would cry because when putting together his obituary, it was difficult for me to digest the fact, I would not write "Ja'Marcus is a 2014 graduate of East Side High School. He attended college at Delta State University majoring in education" since I never thought, I'd be burying my child. My son's life had suddenly ended before it really started. I would never watch my son graduate, but I would watch him receive his high school diploma.

The Diploma

Though this was a major struggle for me, God was still in the mist. Although he did not physically walk across the stage to receive his high school diploma, Mrs. Holmes ensured that Ja'Marcus would know he'd received his diploma. I kept everyone updated on Ja'Marcus' progress on Facebook. During the time he was transitioning, I posted a video of him sucking orange juice out of the sponge. Mrs. Holmes saw the video, and within the hour someone was knocking at my door. After making sure my son was fine, I hurriedly walked down the hallway to see who it was and it was Mrs. Holmes. I asked her to come in and we walked down the hallway to Ja'Marcus' room. I noticed the black object in her hand, but I did not realize it was his diploma. She walked into the room, kissed him on the head and said, "I have something for you." She opened the diploma, handed it to him and asked, "what is this Ja'Marcus?" He looked at her, then down at his diploma and with a low and weak voiced mumbled, "my diploma." Tears of joy fell from his checks as he looked at his name on the diploma. I was joyful as well, but my appreciation for what Mrs. Holmes did will be everlasting.

Ja'Marcus had the worst time trying to pass the History portion of the state exams to graduate. Even during his illness, he went to school to take the History exam. "I think I did good, but I started feeling nauseous" he said after I picked him up. Though I wanted him to pass the test, I knew he was mentally not stable to study effectively to pass it. Mrs. Holmes went above and beyond to help him re-test. She was generous enough to have two East Side staff members come to St. Jude to re-test him. It seemed to always be an obstacle that hindered him. During this time, he'd been diagnosed with Gilliam-

Barre Syndrome. It was difficult for him to hold his pencil, but he managed to do his best. If he'd passed the test I would be thrilled, but if he did not, I would not attack him for it. He was going through too much. I thought he did great for attempting to take the test. However, through it all Mrs. Holmes made sure my son died knowing he had his diploma.

Days before the funeral, his father had audacity to come to my house inquiring about his relative's names being added to the obituary. This was not an issue, but I really could not believe what he was asking me. I stared at him for a minute in total shock, thinking "are you seriously asking me this right now?" This man was concerned about names going in an obituary instead of asking me did I had adequate funds to bury his son! Everything at this point was irrelevant to me. I wanted to call him every name under the sun, but I am so thankful for the Holy Spirit. On the other hand, what made me believe he was going to give me money for his son's funeral expenses, when he's never purchased a bag of pampers or a can of milk? After asking myself those questions, I hurriedly stated "Yes, I have all of your family's information. I contacted your sister via Facebook and she gave me what I needed to complete my son's program." I then opened the door and went in the house. The last thing on earth I wanted was for my son to pass away, but not having to see or converse with his father ever again was the most excellent thing that happened to me in 2014.

The principal of East Side High School, Dr. Randy Grierson was more than amazing. He reached out to me constantly during Ja'Marcus' inpatient hospital visits. He gave me the opportunity to have Ja'Marcus' funeral at the school, and this blessed my soul because Ja'Marcus loved East Side High School. He had a beautiful hand-painted picture of Ja'Marcus designed for me and his constant inspiring words always made my day. Ja'Marcus had been a part of the Cleveland School District for 4 years, but it felt as if he'd been there a lifetime. The love was genuine, and we could feel it.

The Wake

The day of the wake I was in awe at how many people from the community and surrounding areas came to show their support. Many of my Facebook friends were not just clicking "like" on statues, but they demonstrated physical support. This was the first time I met my son's grandmother on his father's side. She had a beautiful spirit and shared a lot of wisdom with me. It was through her I learned that an individual in her family may have had the same illness Ja'Marcus had, but it was never diagnosed. In earlier years, it was difficult to diagnose illnesses since technology was limited. She told me the symptoms that her loved one had and they were identical to my son's. This eased my mind, because I'd learned the **cancer** was linked to a genetic condition. I beat myself up day and night knowing one of us was responsible for my son's death. "This is something neither of you had any control over" are the words the nurse would say to me when I'd tell her that I or his father caused his illness. To this very day, those thoughts still haunt me.

The Funeral

The day of the funeral, I thought I would lose it, but my heart was filled with the spirit. Jesus was surly working in my life and I felt it in my spirit. The support was so great, until I did not have time to shed a tear. I totally recognized once the funeral was over and everyone went their separate ways, the tears was under way. I continued to pray because I did not want to lose my mind or become depressed. I had to be strong for my children, for myself, but most all I needed to be strong for my son. Inwardly I had died, but I needed to live again for him. He never wanted me to worry about him and now I knew he was safe.

As I walked into East Side High School's gymnasium, I looked up and the bleachers were filled. A glad heart is an understatement. At that point, I knew my son's testimony touched many. I smiled as my husband and I gradually walked to the front of the gym, nearly 15 feet away from my son's casket. Looking at his casket gave me an uneasy spirit. I never imagined in life, I would be laying to rest my 18-year-old son. Yes, the physical me was suffering, but my spiritual being was at peace.

Ja'Marcus' funeral was 2 ½ to 3 hours long. I did not intend for it to be this long, but to be honest, I did not want to let go. Funerals are a process that calmly pronounces "the end is nearing." The thoughts of my child being gone greatly suppressed my emotions. I had to stay calm because I did not want my son's funeral to be sad. I believed I set the tone to have a joyful funeral. My son had a home-going celebration. There was more laughter than tears and more smiles than frowns. God was working in a manner like I've never experienced. I wanted to cry, but I could not. God has an amazing way of working huh? My son was lying in his casket right before my eyes, yet I had no desire to cry. This is what happens when God knows you. For anyone can say, "they know God", but the question is does God know you? Having a relationship with God should not begin when you get in a storm, He should already be in your heart. I had to learn this the hard way (chapter 10). I Thessalonian 5:16; teaches us to pray without ceasing and by doing this we prepare ourselves for life's storms in advance. I could not look to my own hope, but to Christ who supplies all hope. Without daily devotions and tears I would not have had the strength to endure this indescribable sorrow.

Ja'Marcus' funeral was satisfying. The singing touched my heart and the kind remarks blessed my soul. There was one part of his celebration that will embrace me for a lifetime. My classmate's son wanted to minister to our hearts in song, but he was not on the obituary. This was not an issue since I immediately gave him the microphone. He wanted to come to the hospital to sing with Ja'Marcus on several occasions, but things were constantly changing. Ja'Marcus loved children and since he was a singer too, this would have been a good experience for them both. This child is the new age Marvin Sapp. He may have been small in stature, but his voice was 6'5. He'd been blessed with a voice that will take you out of this world. He gave me chills when he loudly sang "take me to the king." The thoughts of him singing continues to bless my soul. The Delmar Avenue Inspirational Singers, One in the Spirt and East Side High School Chorus sang their hearts out, but this child received a standing ovation.

The Burial

Darkness had fell as we headed to the burial ground. A countless number of cars followed as we headed to bid my son a farewell. Oftentimes, only family members are preset during the burial, but then I turned around, and my view was astounding. Vehicles filled the dark roads. All I could see were headlights. This is truly the burial of a hero.

As we got closer to the gravesite, I could feel the climax of the end and I was not ready. I wanted to stop the burial and wait until the morrow since night had caught us, but I'd come to close to the breakdown. Then it had finally hit me. Tears began to flow and they would not stop. Crying was never the issue, not being able to stop was. The cool November breeze gave me chills, but this did not stop me from sobbing and watching them throw dirt on top of my son's casket. When they ask the family to go back to their vehicles because this is oftentimes the most difficult part of the funeral, this is defiantly true. My soul died more and more as they tossed dirt on top of my son. I am so thankful this was merely his body, because prayerfully he will someday wake up and be with the Lord.

"Precious in the sight of the Lord is the death of His saints."

Psalms 116:15 (KJV

A Mother's Reflections
Chapter 33

Once my child transitioned I took the time to reflect on our physical and spiritual journey. Being inside the storm was not comfortable. I was repetitively walking into an indefinite world. As I continued to pray and asking God for continued strength, my load became lighter and I was able stay afloat.

There will be times God will place us in uncomfortable situations for our good. These are the areas in our lives where we may need to be strengthen. God is also teaching us to completely rely on His authority, understanding and comfort. I learned I cannot do anything on my own. Although there will be earthly resources, nothing shall be made possible without our spiritual resource. We need Christ! For us to be where God will have us, we must be willing to step out of our comfort zone. This is not an easy task, but we must be confidant God will give us all we need to prosper.

My journey was a matter of faith and focus. I understood the word of God, but now the time had come for me to use what I'd been taught. Psalm 23 helped me to sincerely put God first regardless of the after effect. One of my favorite scriptures is Psalm 23:1; "the Lord is my shepherd, I shall not want." This is a powerful scripture. It shows us the Lord is the head of our lives. It was because of this verse I could give all my burdens to Christ without doubting for I had built a solid relationship with Christ. David was focused on "walking through the valley." Not once did he say, "If I get through the valley." He recognized he could make it for he knew who was before him. If David could walk through the valley of the shadow of death with no fear, we can do the same. God hasn't given us a spirit of fear... (II Timothy 1:7). God will take us through a storm and we will walk out without a spot, wrinkle or blemish. This may sound easy, but it is a process of focusing, waiting, listening and obeying God. These four things are essential during a storm.

I was bombarded with undesirable thoughts day after day, but I agreed to let the word of God beat the devil, and He worked everything out on my behalf. Believing and trusting in God some days seemed difficult to do but being truly grounded in the word gave me understanding that surpasses all comprehension. God had placed me in a situation where only He could help me out of. I was thankful for such a great support system, but this was a battle that was designed for me, my son and The Lord. God wanted my full attention, therefore, I needed to humble myself and allow Him to be my guide.

It is easy to say, "I am a Christian" when the sea is calm, and the sun is shining, but when the wind begins to blow, and the rain starts to pour; what will you do? Do you have the strength to weather the storm? Many choose to complain, have doubts, run, throw pity parties and even give up. The devil now rejoices, since he believes he has entangled your mind with doubts while you are at your lowest point. Remember, the devil hears your prayers, and there is no time for unwavering faith. You must stand boldly against Satan and show him who your faith is in. If you want to please God, you must have faith (Hebrews 11:6). God is not moved by emotions, but by faith only.

Before God allows us to step into a storm, He knows there is something good on the other side, but we must stay on the boat. If we get out of the boat, we will drown. God is the ship; therefore, we must hold on to His word to keep from losing hope. We can choose to sink into hopelessness or we can hold God's hand through the storm. I oftentimes would say, "God knows the outcome of the storm, we must be patient and wait on His timing." Being patient is key, because your situation will not instantaneously fade away. There will be mountains to climb and deep curves in the road but be of good cheer. God is merely preparing you for a greater you. God always has a better purpose for our lives, than we have for ourselves, but we must be ready and willing to wait on Him.

You may be going through a storm right now. The clouds may be dark, and you can barely see the road, but don't give up. You can make it through! Don't ask God to move your mountain, pray for the strength to climb. While climbing the mountain, you will have cuts, scrapes and bruises. You'll sometimes fall but keep moving and allow Jesus to be the cornerstone in your life. Your adversary, the devil will surly throw fiery darts of doubts your way, but it is your job as a child of God to obey, trust, and have faith in Him. Do you recall in Matthew 14:22-36 when Jesus walked on water? This story is when the disciples were on the Sea of Galilee and a storm came upon them. After Jesus dismissed the crowd, he went up to the mountain to pray. The boat was not only fighting a strong headwind, as it was being beaten by the waves, but it was a far away from land. We know naturally the disciples were praying, but Jesus did not come after hearing their initial supplication. It wasn't until early the next morning he came to them. This helps us to recognize God is always with us. He doesn't come when we want Him too, He comes on His own timing.

After Jesus told Peter who He was, Peter needed confirmation. He then asked Jesus to order him to come on the water with him and Jesus replied "come" and once Peter begin to walk on water, he began to sink. Why did Peter sink? He lacked faith. Many of us can relate to this passage of scripture. God has revealed Himself to us on several occasions, but we still need confirmation. We've walked into uncertain situations plenty of times and God has always been there. Once Peter started walking on water, he took his eyes off Jesus, as we do when it seems our lives are perfect. Regardless of how good things may be going in our life, we should always keep our eyes on Him.

My Big Mama use to say, "life isn't easy, but it is fair." I didn't understand that statement until I was much older. and I agree, she was right. God never promised us an easy life, but He did promise to never leave or forsake us (Deuteronomy 31:6). As you read in chapter 10, my faith was tested, and I failed. Why? I was not genuine to God, but to my own selfish ways. Going to church means nothing, if your heart isn't sincere. Singing, clapping, and using those so-called holy cliques won't cut it. For every song, you sing and "amen and hallelujahs" your utter, God will test. I learned a treasured lesson during my storm. God is not the man to play with. We can front for man. We can even mislead ourselves, but we cannot deceive God. If you haven't been in a storm, keep living. Your storm is brewing but be of good cheer. Like me, you can overcome.

Although my son died from **cancer** physically, spiritually he yet lives. My hope for others is to kick **cancer's** butt and physically live.

May the God of hope fill you with all joy and peace as you trust in him, so that you may overflow with hope by the power of the Holy Spirit.

Rom. 15:13 (NIV

Although my son's physical journey on earth was short-lived. His Christlike attributes will endure endlessly in the countless number of hearts he impressed.

#Joy4Jayy

Made in the USA
Columbia, SC
12 February 2023